Simone.

INTEN

GW00372676

MODERN NURSING SERIES

General Editors
SUSAN E NORMAN, SRN, NDN Cert, RNT
Senior Tutor, The Nightingale School, West Lambeth Health Authority

JEAN HEATH, BA, SRN, SCM, Cert Ed
National Health Learning Resources Unit, Sheffield City Polytechnic

Consultant Editor
A J HARDING RAINS, MS, FRCS
Regional Dean, British Postgraduate Medical Federation;
formerly Professor of Surgery, Charing Cross Hospital Medical School;
Honorary Consultant Surgeon, Charing Cross Hospital;
Honorary Consultant Surgeon to the Army

This Series caters for the needs of a wide range of nursing, medical and ancillary professions. Some of the titles are given below, but a complete list is available from the Publisher.

General Surgery and the Nurse
R E HORTON

Principles of Surgery and Surgical Nursing
SELWYN TAYLOR

Neurology
EDWIN R BICKERSTAFF

Nursing—Image or Reality?
MARGARET C SCHURR and JANET TURNER

Community Child Health
MARION E JEPSON

Gerontology and Geriatric Nursing
SIR W FERGUSON ANDERSON, F I CAIRD, R D KENNEDY and DORIS SCHWARTZ

Taverner's Physiology
DERYCK TAVERNER

INTENSIVE CARE

A K Yates
MB, ChB, FRCS
Consultant Cardiothoracic Surgeon, Guy's Hospital, London;
Director, Cardiothoracic Unit and Consultant in Charge,
Surgical Intensive Care Unit, Guy's Hospital, London

P J Moorhead
MB, ChB, MRCP
Consultant Physician, Northern General Hospital, Sheffield

A P Adams
PhD, MB, BS, FFARCS
Professor of Anaesthetics in the University of London at the United
Medical and Dental Schools of Guy's and St Thomas' Hospitals;
Head of Department of Anaesthetics and Honorary Consultant Anaesthetist,
Guy's Hospital, London

HODDER AND STOUGHTON
LONDON SYDNEY AUCKLAND TORONTO

The cover photograph was taken in the Critical Care Unit at St. Göran's Hospital in Stockholm by Engström Medical AB of Sweden, and is reproduced with the kind permission of LKB Instruments Ltd.

British Library Cataloguing in Publication Data

Yates, A. K.
    Intensive care.—(Modern nursing series)
    1. Critical care medicine
    I. Title   II. Moorhead, P. J.
    III. Adams, A. P.   IV. Series
    616'028   RC86.7
    ISBN 0 340 33113 5

First printed 1984

Photo Typeset by Macmillan India Ltd., Bangalore

Printed in Great Britain
for Hodder and Stoughton Educational
a division of Hodder and Stoughton Ltd.,
Mill Road, Dunton Green, Sevenoaks, Kent,
by Biddles Ltd, Guildford, Surrey

Editors' Foreword

This well established series of books reflects contemporary nursing and health care practice. It is used by a wide range of nursing, medical and ancillary professions and encompasses titles suitable for different levels of experience from those in training to those who have qualified.

Members of the nursing professions need to be highly informed and to keep critically abreast of demanding changes in attitudes and technology. The series therefore continues to grow with new titles being added to the list and existing titles being updated regularly. Its aim is to promote sound understanding by presenting essential facts clearly and concisely. We hope this will lead to nursing care of the highest standard.

Preface

Intensive care is a speciality which demands an understanding of all aspects of clinical medicine and their application to the critically ill patient. Continuing developments in medical research and technology have made it a highly skilled subject for the nurses, doctors and technicians involved, for whom this book is written.

The purpose of intensive care is to monitor, control and support the failing vital functions of the body. Derangement of one biological system may lead to complications in the others, hence care of the patient requires a detailed and integrated knowledge of the functions of the body in both normal and abnormal situations. This book considers each biological system separately so that the basic underlying theoretical and practical principles may be easily appreciated and intelligently applied.

Intensive Care Units vary widely in their scope; some are primarily concerned with patients admitted after operation (e.g. after cardio-pulmonary bypass), others with patients suffering from severe respiratory disease such as intractable asthma, others with problems presented by patients who are victims of road traffic accidents with multiple injuries or who have attempted suicide. Whatever the nature of the trauma or the disease process, Intensive Care Units demand team work and discipline of the highest order. We hope that this book will be welcomed by all members of the intensive care team.

A K Yates
P J Moorhead
A P Adams
1983

Intensive Care has evolved from an earlier publication, 'Principles of Intensive Care', in response to the considerable changes in practice and technique over the last decade. We would like to express our thanks for the contributions made by Dr D. B. Jeffreys of Guy's Hospital to *Poisoning* (Chapter 6) and Miss Diana Caulfeild-Stoker SRN of Guy's Hospital to *Nursing Care and Procedures* (Chapter 10).

Acknowledgements

The publisher wishes to acknowledge the following for granting permission to reprint their material in this book:

Dr Penelope Bolton Hewitt, Department of Anaesthetics, Guy's Hospital, for devising the Neurological Observation Chart, *Appendix VI*; Franklin Scientific Publications Ltd. for **Figs. 2.18, 3.2 & 3.3** (from *Principles and Practice of Blood-Gas Analysis* by A. P. Adams and C. E. W. Hahn); The Chartered Society of Physiotherapy for **Figs. 2.19 (a), (b), (c) & 7.2** (from *Physiotherapy, 66,* no. 5, 1980 and *58,* p. 275, 1972); American Edwards Laboratories for **Figs. 2.22 (a) & (b)** (Swan-Ganz is a registered trademark of the American Edwards Laboratories); Dr E. R. Bickerstaff for **Figs. 7.1 & 7.4** (from *Neurology,* Modern Nursing Series): the editors of *Anesthesiology* for **Figs. 7.5 & 7.10** (from *Anesthesiology, 47,* nos. 2 & 4, Aug. 1977); Northwood Publications Ltd. for **Figs. 7.7 & 7.8** (from *British Journal of Clinical Equipment,* May 1980, D. J. Price); Miss V. Mielton, Chief Dietician, Guy's Hospital for **Table 9.2**; the editors of *British Medical Journal* for the extract on p. 158 from the article 'Diagnosis of Brain Death', 1976, *ii,* 1069–70.

Contents

1

General Considerations

The care of the individual patient in the Intensive Care Unit (ICU) demands team work of the highest order. It requires good administrative ability as well as tact and good relationships between colleagues, both medical and nursing. Above all the patient must receive the best medical attention and medical politics must never be allowed to interfere with this aim.

One doctor of consultant status should be in charge of the unit, and he must be trusted by his colleagues and given considerable authority in the management of the unit. Intensive care is gradually becoming a speciality in its own right, and anaesthetists are playing a major part in the establishment and organisation of units. The modern anaesthetist is well trained in the management of physiological disturbances and his specialised knowledge of respiratory physiology and ventilator management makes him a particularly suitable choice. The nature and training of their speciality plus the anaesthetists' impartiality regarding bed designation make them suitable to administrate such a unit. Many units, however, prefer a surgeon or physician to fill this role. It is important that the person in charge has an enthusiastic interest in this aspect of medicine, and has the tact and skill to work well as the leader of the team. Even if an anaesthetist is not in charge, he should be an important member of an intensive care team. He and his junior colleagues are invaluable for respiratory support and technical skills such as intubation and ventilation.

The intensive care team should not be too large so that continuity of patient care may be preserved, and relevant experts of other disciplines should be consulted to deal with specific problems only as they arise. It is desirable to have an Intensive Care Committee which allows members of the team to be represented along with other interested members of the hospital staff when important decisions are being formulated.

Patient responsibility

The responsibility for the patient's treatment should generally rest with the consultant under whom the patient was admitted to the hospital in the first place. Treatment will normally be initiated by house officers and registrars who play an important part in the work of the unit. The consultant in charge of the unit will liaise to ensure that optimal treatment is given and that the patient is discharged when intensive care is no longer required. The consultant in charge of the unit will also have control over admissions, although it may be that only difficult decisions are referred to him.

As the hospital junior staff play such an important part in the running of the unit, it is important that they should be involved in rounds and discussions. The clinical condition of patients needing intensive care demands close observation and full and accurate communication between members of the team. Each unit develops its own system, but one routine business round per day including all the involved personnel is advisable. This ensures an integrated and organised programme of care. There should be at least one anaesthetist immediately available 24 hours per day in the unit.

Planning and organisation

No universally ideal plan for an ICU exists, and it will vary according to the requirements of the unit and the space and staff available. A general layout is illustrated in Fig. 1.1.

The fixed Central Nursing Station is probably not the best method of observation except in the Coronary Care Unit where patients should be nursed in a quiet atmosphere. Automatic recording of vital parameters, such as the electrocardiogram (ECG) and vascular pressure, and the making of patients' records by means of trend recorders can be done at the central station. In general the nurse should not be remote from the patient and, if staffing permits, the best system is where the nurse is at the bedside, aided by the bedside monitor and not replaced by it. Even where nurses are scarce, one good nurse working in a room with as many as four patients is better than the same nurse sitting at a central station watching from afar.

The Coronary Care Unit is best separated from the ICU to ensure that coronary patients are not disturbed by the noise and drama sometimes associated with the general ICU.

The size of the unit depends upon two factors—the size of the hospital and the type of patients receiving treatment in the hospital. In hospitals with thoracic or neurosurgical units, the proportion of beds allocated to intensive care will be higher than in a general hospital. Figures between 1% (or less) and 4% have been quoted—the larger for the hospital carrying out highly specialised operations, and the lower figure for the general hospital. There must be at least four beds to merit the staffing and organisation of such a unit.

It is equally important that the ICU should not be too large and unwieldy. Its use should not be encouraged for patients who do not strictly need intensive care. Rather than an oversize unit, several smaller sections such as coronary care, renal and surgical ICUs are preferred. It is unwise to combine recovery wards with intensive care, unless this is dictated by space and financial considerations. Postoperative cases may qualify for admission and will then be transferred from recovery to the unit.

No new acute hospital should be built without an ICU and modern planning allows previous mistakes to be avoided. Plans which involve the lack of provision for natural light must be resisted. In general, cubicles are best for infected patients or those requiring treatment by dialysis as there is good evidence that this will prevent cross infection.

Rather than physically separating the sub-sections of intensive care, it is better to divide off one large area for the several purposes. This allows increased flexibility of staff, simplification of administration, and avoids duplication of expensive equipment.

A busy ICU needs at least four staff nurses for each bed. This allows for sickness, lectures, off-duty and holidays. In addition, sisters must be present in sufficient numbers to cover night as well as day duty. Sisters lend stability to the unit, and one of them should be designated 'In Charge'. The nurse complement will be of varying seniority. Some will be senior and experienced in intensive care having completed a course; others will be working while on the course. It is desirable that student nurses should also attend the unit as part of their training.

The use of larger open areas will reduce the work load on the nursing staff. Infective patients will require especial care and these generally fall into three groups:

1 potentially infective cases, e.g. tracheostomy;
2 frankly infective cases, e.g. faecal fistula, open suppuration;
3 immuno-suppressed patients, e.g. following renal transplant.

Group 1 is best treated in single rooms, but patients belonging to Groups 2 and 3 should be treated in isolation. This should be a specially designated section. Isolation rooms must have proper barrier precautions and separate nurses if possible. Nurses can be dressed in different coloured dresses to distinguish them. Ideally they should not mix with nurses from the 'clean' areas while on duty.

The shape of the unit is to some extent immaterial and will be dictated by the building. For the frankly infective patients there will be either a 'dirty' unit adjacent to the main unit or an isolation room at the end of the unit. This would be at the distal end of the ventilation route. Ideally the main operating theatre should be in close proximity to the unit. If this is not so, it may be wise to have a small theatre in the ICU. This is particularly important if the hospital is engaged in open-heart surgery, where a long journey back to the operating theatre could jeopardise the chances of survival. The theatre could also be used for other operations such as tracheostomy and insertion of pacemakers.

A twenty-four hour biochemical laboratory service is essential. Blood gas analysis should be available in a laboratory in the unit at all times. The equipment should ideally be maintained and operated by technicians.

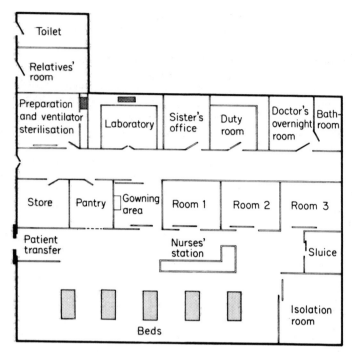

Fig. 1.1 An eight bed Intensive Care Unit. More than one relatives' room is desirable and these should not be along the main route of entry/exit to the unit. There should be as much space as possible for storage; many units have been built with insufficient storage space. Day rooms where medical, nursing and technical staff may relax for coffee etc. are very important and should be provided with windows and a pleasant outlook

Although modern automated equipment can be operated by non-technical staff, a technical 'back-up' service is essential to guarantee quality control of samples analysed.

Technical assistance should be available for maintaining electronic equipment, also on a 24 hour basis.

Clothing. Full barrier techniques must be observed when nursing patients in designated isolation rooms. It is emphasised that any relaxation of barrier nursing invalidates its function and demoralises the attendant nursing staff. It is not uncommon for visiting doctors to ignore a barrier system and it is important that all erring personnel are immediately corrected.

In the other ICU areas it is generally recognised that it is unnecessary to wear special clothing as any such system is never comprehensively applied; as well as having no proven benefit, its haphazard application devalues the importance and impairs the practice of complete barrier nursing in septic and immuno-suppressed patients. One unit requires that people entering the patients' area of the unit simply remove their coats and this policy is an effective way of dissuading entry by those who have no good reason to be there.

Entrance. The entrance to the unit should be a double-door air lock. One door will not open unless the other door is closed. Facilities for washing and changing should be situated at the entrance.

Ventilation and heating. These should be of modern standards with 5 micrometer (μm) filtration and positive pressure ventilation. The air flow should be from the 'clean' to the 'dirtier' end of the unit. Humidity and temperature should be controlled. Staff toilets should be outside the 'clean' section of the unit. Kitchen facilities are required as part of the unit.

Piped gases. These should be available and Entonox (50% nitrous oxide and oxygen mixture) is useful in addition to oxygen and medical (oil-free) air, which are essential.

Suction. Piped suction with low and high pressure outlets must be available at every bed space.

Lighting. This should be colour-corrected to assist in clinical assessment of skin colour. Colour-corrected fluorescent tubes emit less light than ordinary commercial tubes, so an adequate number of fluorescent lights and hence a suitable intensity of illumination should be determined. Dim lighting should be available for night use. Anglepoise lighting is useful at the bedside, and a theatre-type spotlight for emergency procedures such as tracheostomy.

Power points. These should be plentiful and they should be placed at the bedside and at strategic places around the rooms. They will of course be required in the ancillary rooms such as preparation rooms and storage rooms.

Visitors. These should be restricted to the nearest relatives. Surgical patients in particular should have a minimum of visitors. Visitors must change to the same degree as medical personnel. Overnight accommodation should be available for relatives of the seriously ill.

Flowers. These should not be allowed in the 'clean' section of the ward, but can be viewed through the glass where possible.

Patients' transfer zone. This should be as in an operating theatre with transfer to a clean trolley or bed.

The hospital *bacteriologist* should be involved in sterilisation procedures and the standard of ward cleaning. Frequent nasal swabs should be taken from the unit staff. Sink drains can be treated each week by the careful use of sodium hydroxide pellets BP (97.5% sodium hydroxide) and 10% formaldehyde.

The unit should contain rooms for storage of equipment and sterilisation, a workshop, preparation rooms, offices and day rooms for nurses and doctors. Lockers must be available for patients' and nurses' valuables.

Ideally each bed should have monitoring oscilloscopes to permit the ready display of vital waveforms and digital values related to these. A resuscitation trolley must always be available in the ward, fully equipped and checked daily. A defibrillator and pacemaker must also be available at all times.

The design of beds is always under discussion. Ideally they should tip at both ends, with an adjustment for height. They should be mobile and under-mattress boards must be available. Easy access to the head of the patient to permit nursing and medical procedures is essential. Monitoring and life-support equipment with their associated cables and tubes should also be positioned carefully to avoid accidents and to permit patient access.

2

The Cardiovascular System

The normal circulation

The rhythm of the healthy heart is termed sinus rhythm. This is a synchronised myocardial contraction, the cycle commencing with right and left atrial contraction pumping the blood, at low pressure, into the ventricles to 'prime' them. This phase is termed *diastole*. Subsequently the ventricles eject this blood into the great arteries during *systole*.

The physiological range of cardiovascular function is very large. The normal heart rate can range from 40–180 beats per minute depending on the fitness, age and activity of the person. The cardiac output of blood has an equally impressive range from about 4 litres per minute at rest to 19–37 litres per minute during strenuous exercise. This is more conveniently expressed as the *cardiac index* which is the cardiac output (in litres per minute) divided by the surface area of the body (in square metres). The cardiac index is independent of the size of the individual and is usually about 3 at rest.

The work done by the heart is related to:

    (i) the volume of blood ejected by the ventricles;
    (ii) the resistance to the ejection of this blood which, in the absence of valve stenosis, is termed the peripheral resistance.

The blood flows in sequence from the systemic veins to the right heart then through the lungs to the left heart and from the left heart to the systemic arterial system to complete the circuit. The right ventricle must therefore eject the same volume of blood as the left ventricle. The peripheral resistance to blood flow through the pulmonary vascular bed is approximately one quarter of the peripheral resistance of the systemic vascular bed and this is why the right ventricular pressures (normal 18–30 mmHg or 2.4–4.0 kPa systolic and −2 to 2 mmHg or −0.3–0.3 kPa diastolic) and pulmonary artery pressures (normal 18–30 mmHg or 2.4–4.0 kPa systolic and 0.9–1.6 kPa diastolic) are much lower than the left ventricular and systemic arterial pressures. These pressure differences reflect the less work done by the right compared to the left ventricle although they maintain an equal output.

Normal function of the body depends on the healthy function of the individual cells. The cardiovascular system is a servo-mechanism transporting oxygen, food, water, electrolytes, hormones, defence cells and antibodies to the tissues, and metabolic breakdown products (e.g. urea and carbon dioxide) and heat away from the cells.

In the short term the most important function is *oxygen transport*. If the circulation arrests at normal body temperature irreversible brain damage occurs within five minutes because of anoxia. If the circulation is sub-optimal then all the functions are embarrassed; if this unsatisfactory state of affairs continues there is progressive cell and therefore organ failure and finally death. In circulatory failure the organs most rapidly affected are the brain, kidneys, lungs and heart.

A satisfactory circulation depends on many factors:

1   Adequate blood volume

The blood volume in an average adult of 70 kilograms is approximately 5 litres. This can be conveniently expressed as about 2.8 litres per square metre of body surface area or 70 ml per kilogram body weight. The blood volume is 80–85 ml/kg in the newborn, 75 ml/kg between six weeks and two years and 72 ml/kg between two years and puberty.

2   Adequate oxygen carrying power of the blood

This depends on a normal haemoglobin content. In the adult the normal range of haemoglobin is 12–16 g/100 ml of blood and it is contained in the red blood cells (erythrocytes). At birth the normal range is higher, being 18–27 g/100 ml of blood. This progressively falls to 9–15 g/100 ml by the age of one year and then progressively rises until reaching the adult range by puberty. In the female, haemoglobin levels tend to be lower than in men. The normal range of the erythrocyte count is 4.5–6 million cells per mm^3 of blood, being rather higher in the newborn. These cells make up approximately 46% of the blood volume, this value being known as the *haematocrit*.

3   Satisfactory oxygen content of the blood

In the healthy person this depends on adequate respiratory function, which is discussed in Chapter 3. Normally arterial blood is over 95% saturated, giving an oxygen content of about 20 ml in each 100 ml of blood.

4   Satisfactory myocardial contractility

The heart muscle contracts at differing speed and force in health, such that it ejects all the blood that enters it. Any impairment in contraction, from whatever cause, will reduce the cardiac output.

Factors that may cause cardiovascular failure

  1 Abnormal blood volume
     (a) hypovolaemia
     (b) hypervolaemia

2 Inadequate oxygen carrying power
3 Inadequate oxygen content
4 Inadequate myocardial contractility
    (a) direct myocardial damage due to local anoxia, toxins (chemical, bacterial)
    (b) valve dysfunction due to rheumatic fever, bacterial endocarditis, viral or fungal endocarditis, degenerative causes, congenital causes
    (c) general inadequate tissue oxygenation
    (d) dysrhythmias
    (e) tamponade or constriction of the heart
    (f) electrolyte imbalance
    (g) acid-base imbalance
5 Humoral imbalance
6 Obstructed circulation

These will now be dealt with in detail.

Abnormal blood volume

Hypovolaemia and the value of central venous pressure (CVP) measurement

If the blood volume falls below normal, the arterial volume is maintained at the expense of the venous volume. The first indication of a low blood volume is a low central venous pressure (normal range $0-5\,cmH_2O$ or $0-0.5\,kPa$)*. Because the reduced blood volume must be circulated more rapidly to maintain the same rate of oxygen delivery to the tissues, there is a tachycardia. The arterial pressure remains within the normal range until the hypovolaemia is severe enough to cause decompensation of the cardiovascular system.

The cardinal sign of hypovolaemia is therefore a low CVP and one should not wait for a tachycardia or a falling blood pressure before initiating treatment. Hypovolaemia is commonly said to be obvious; this is in fact true only when haemorrhage is external and therefore 'obvious'. Most of the classically described signs of acute hypovolaemia (pallor, sweating, low blood pressure, small pulse pressure, cold extremities and restlessness) are the signs of an inadequate cardiac output and may be precipitated by any acute catastrophe not necessarily associated with hypovolaemia.

* The use of cmH_2O is popular in units where measurements are made using a column of saline. Some people prefer to use units of mmHg; since the density of mercury is 13.6 times greater than that of water or saline, $10\,cmH_2O = 7.35\,mmHg$ (NB $1\,kPa = 7.5\,mmHg$).

A low central venous pressure determines the diagnosis of hypovolaemia; the other observations relate to the low cardiac output. Appreciation of this fact is of the utmost importance in the shocked patient who has a totally concealed haemorrhage. It is even more so in less acutely developing hypovolaemia, when even the 'typical' signs are not obvious.

In conditions of cardiovascular stress or failure, from whatever cause, accurate monitoring of the CVP is essential. Except in cases of right or left 'congestive' ventricular failure and tamponade, when the CVP will already be high, raising the pressure to 5–15 cmH$_2$O (0.5–1.5 kPa) is always beneficial. The danger of over-transfusion during this procedure is completely obviated by the very fact that the CVP is being monitored. It is difficult to overstate the importance of accurate monitoring of the CVP. If the pressure is held at 5–15 cmH$_2$O one can be sure that the blood volume is adequate. It is certainly the most valuable method of ensuring adequate blood replacement in conditions of haemorrhage, being superior to direct volumetric measurement of blood loss, blood volume measurements and patient weighing techniques (Fig. 2.1). The CVP is also valuable in the assessment of general body hydration. It will always be low (zero or lower) in cases of dehydration.

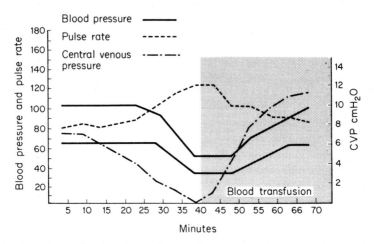

Fig. 2.1 Charts showing the cardiovascular response to an acute haemorrhage with subsequent blood transfusion raising the CVP to 12 cmH$_2$O. Blood replacement is related to the CVP and not to the measured blood loss. Note that a falling venous pressure is the first indication of hypovolaemia

A patient in shock due to causes other than haemorrhage or dehydration will have a normal blood volume, but a significant proportion of this volume may become sequestered from the circulation, probably becoming pooled in an abnormally dilated visceral vascular bed. This condition of functional hypovolaemia has been descriptively termed 'intravascular haemorrhage' and is associated with a low CVP, requiring treatment. In this common condition blood volume expanders such as dextran or plasma should be used to raise the CVP to optimal levels.

An accurate CVP manometer will always reveal hypovolaemia except in the occasional case of the hypovolaemic patient who has been incorrectly treated solely by vasoconstrictor drugs such as adrenaline. The resulting intense arterial and venous spasm can artificially maintain the venous pressure at normal levels. The CVP will not be raised above normal in these circumstances and applying the '5 to 15 rule' will ensure this pitfall is avoided. In many cases it is surprising how much fluid must be transfused before the CVP begins to rise. It is of course important to be sure that the tip of the CVP catheter is indeed in the 'central' position— that is, in a great vein within the chest or in the right atrium. The position is checked by X-ray and by observing 'swings' in the column of fluid during respiration.

In summary it can be stated that setting up an accurate CVP monitoring system is one of the immediate priorities in the intensive care of a patient. If the venous pressure is less than $5\,cmH_2O$ (0.5 kPa) the blood volume should be expanded to raise the pressure to the order of $5\,cmH_2O$. While intravenous fluids are being given to expand the blood volume, the other parameters indicating the patient's cardiac output (see page 41) are closely observed. The optimal CVP level in each individual case will be that level at which maximum cardiovascular response is gained. Usually this is in the range of $8-12\,cmH_2O$ (0.8–1.2 kPa). The fluid indicated to expand the blood volume will depend on the exact circumstances at the time: blood if there is haemorrhage; packed red blood cells in anaemia; electrolyte solutions if there is water or salt depletion and non-haemic blood expanders in the condition of intra-vascular sequestration. This management ensures that:

(i) concealed hypovolaemia is not present;
(ii) the heart has a strong physiological drive by ensuring adequate filling of the cardiac chambers;
(iii) myocardial congestive failure or constriction is immediately indicated by the high venous pressure if and when it occurs;
(iv) there is a valuable indication of response to treatment.

It is important to stress that in any patient with the signs of low cardiac output and who has a low CVP one should never be discouraged by the sometimes alarming volume of fluid required to raise the venous pressure. Only when the circulatory system is full will the venous pressure begin to rise and sometimes 1–2 litres must be given before this state of affairs is reached. Once the circulatory system is full only small volumes of fluid are then necessary to maintain the venous pressure at the desired level. By far the commonest sub-optimal treatment in cardiovascular failure is inadequate expansion of the blood volume.

Hypervolaemia

This is usually associated with excessive transfusion. It will not occur if intravenous transfusions of significant volume are monitored by CVP. The risk is greatest in the elderly and the very young.

The first indication of hypervolaemia is a venous pressure rising to an abnormally high level which is, for practical purposes, above 15 cmH$_2$O (1.5 kPa). At pressures above this level pulmonary oedema or peripheral congestion may occur. In hypervolaemia there is a progressive build up of blood in the venous side of the circulation. Pulmonary venous congestion and oedema impair oxygenation of the blood and increasing dyspnoea ensues with decreasing oxygen transport. This results in the vicious circle of hypoxia leading to a reduced cardiac output. In general the right atrial (RA) pressure changes in the same manner as the left atrial (LA) pressure, even in cases of 'isolated' left ventricular failure, e.g. myocardial infarction. The absolute levels may not be the same but the trend is the same. In right and left atrial catheterised patients after left heart operations an LA pressure more than the order of 10 cmH$_2$O (1.0 kPa) higher than the RA pressure has not been observed. If the RA pressure is not allowed to rise above 15 cmH$_2$O the risk of pulmonary oedema is avoided. These comments are valid only in the presence of a competent mitral valve.

If the venous pressure is at danger level any transfusion should be stopped, intravenous diuretics given and in acute and severe cases with frank pulmonary oedema phlebotomy may even be performed to lower the CVP rapidly. It should be noted that if over-transfusion or myocardial failure does precipitate pulmonary oedema, the measures utilised to reduce the CVP should not lower it to abnormally low levels, i.e. below 5 cmH$_2$O, otherwise the cardiac failure may be increased due to relative hypovolaemia.

It is strongly recommended that whenever it is intended to administer significant volumes of intravenous fluids, a central catheter should be utilised to monitor CVP. It is suggested that all critically ill patients with cardiovascular instability warrant optimum monitoring of the heart and in this respect the LA pressure should be monitored as well as the CVP (RA pressure). The LA pressure can be indirectly monitored relatively easily by insertion of a Swan-Ganz catheter (see page 50). This allows even more accurate assessment of cardiac function.

Inadequate oxygen carrying power

This is usually related to anaemia. For clinical purposes the anaemias may be classified into three groups, each of which has many subdivisions:

  (i) *post-haemorrhagic anaemia*, following haemorrhage;
  (ii) *aregenerative anaemia*, resulting from deficient bone marrow function;

(iii) *haemolytic anaemia*, resulting from excessive destruction of red blood corpuscles.

Any anaemia can be corrected in the short term by blood transfusion. In the long term, treatment depends on identification of the type of anaemia and specific treatment of the cause. This is not within the terms of reference of intensive care. Exceptionally, a satisfactory haemoglobin level is rendered non-functional with regard to oxygen transport, as in the case of carbon monoxide poisoning.

In conditions of cardiovascular stress it is important to maintain an adequate haemoglobin level to ensure that as much oxygen as possible is delivered to the tissues. Haemoglobin and haematocrit estimations are important and these should be checked regularly during the period of intensive care. If anaemia is present it should be corrected as soon as possible by transfusion of freshly packed red blood cells. Hypoxia in conjunction with cardiovascular failure is a common and important cause of progressive deterioration and every step should be taken to avoid this. It is so important to maintain good oxygen transport that, if anaemia exists, red cell transfusion should be given, even in the presence of congestive cardiac failure. In these cases packed red blood cells are given slowly, each unit being covered by preliminary intravenous injection of a diuretic (e.g. frusemide, 20 mg) coupled with accurate monitoring of the CVP.

A rough estimate of the required volume of packed cells can be made if the patient's blood volume is assessed (3 litres per square metre of surface area; 70 ml/kg body weight), the haemoglobin content of one unit of blood being 35–50 g. In the average adult of 70 kg transfusion of one 500 ml unit of blood will raise the haemoglobin content by approximately 1 g/100 ml of blood.

When considering the optimum haemoglobin level in a patient with low cardiac output it should be appreciated that there is a balance between the oxygen carrying power of the blood (haemoglobin level) and the blood viscosity (which rises with increasing haemoglobin level). Increasing blood viscosity impairs capillary blood flow. It is generally accepted that, provided cardiac output and full saturation of haemoglobin with oxygen and blood volume are maintained, a haematocrit as low as 30 % (Hb 10 g/100 ml) is of no disadvantage in reference to tissue perfusion and oxygenation because the reduced oxygen carrying power is 'counter-balanced' by the reduced viscosity of the blood, enhancing capillary flow and oxygenation.

Inadequate oxygen content

If the venous blood is not fully oxygenated during its passage through the lungs, or partially bypasses the lungs due to a congenital abnormality, such as Tetralogy of Fallot, the oxygen tension and the oxygen content of the arterial blood will be below normal. If the arterial oxygen tension remains below values of about 60–70 mmHg (7.98–9.31 kPa) progressively significant tissue hypoxia develops.

In anatomical right-to-left shunts due to congenital cyanotic heart disease the long term tissue hypoxia results in polycythaemia with high haemoglobin and haematocrit, the haemoglobin often rising above 20 g/100 ml of blood. This raises the total oxygen carrying power per unit of blood and as a result the volume of contained oxygen for a given oxygen tension will be greater. The correct management in these conditions is to correct or alleviate the effect of the shunt by operative means. The patient with cyanotic heart disease who is in cardiovascular failure may need admission to the ICU for the purpose of improving the cardiac function before embarking on an operation. In these cases it is important to maintain a high inspiratory oxygen concentration, good respiratory function and to maintain the high haemoglobin content of the blood. This ensures as high a tissue oxygenation as possible. It is fundamentally incorrect to attempt to reduce the abnormally high haemoglobin and haematocrit of these patients, unless it is in conjunction with an operation which will effectively reduce or stop the detrimental effect of the shunt.

By far the commonest cause of arterial oxygen desaturation is perfusion/ventilation imbalance in the lungs (page 64). Normally a small proportion of the blood flowing through the lungs does not come into contact with a respiratory alveolar surface and therefore is not able to take up oxygen. This is known as the physiological shunt. In pathological states of the lungs such as consolidation or atelectasis this type of shunt can become large and very significant. Its features and treatment are considered in Chapter 3. Other respiratory causes of inadequate arterial oxygen content including inadequate oxygen content of inspired air and inadequate lung aeration are also considered in this chapter.

Unsatisfactory myocardial contractility

(a)   Direct myocardial damage

Direct myocardial damage commonly arises from coronary artery occlusion by thrombosis or embolism. Bacterial toxins can also produce cellular myocardial damage and this may be due to circulating toxins (toxaemia) as in typhoid fever, or due to circulating living bacteria as in Gram-negative septicaemia. Chemicals, such as alcohol, introduced into the body may also produce toxic myocardial damage.

The myocardial damage may be of varying degree and may be reversible or irreversible. Localised myocardial anoxia will cause increasing irreversible damage at normal body temperature after approximately

30–40 minutes, and an area of ischaemic cardiac muscle will show progressive infarction unless satisfactory coronary blood flow is re-established to the affected area within this time period. There is progressive intracellular vacuolisation, mitochondrial breakdown, loss of potassium and increase of sodium and water. These changes are associated with disruption of the intracellular enzyme systems, i.e. cellular death.

As the myocardial power weakens, the cardiac output and therefore oxygen delivery to the tissues is impaired, with increasing pooling of blood in the venous systems. The decreasing blood flow affects the myocardium as well as the rest of the body. The resulting myocardial hypoxia will aggravate the myocardial condition and a vicious circle is established which, unless broken, will progress to circulatory arrest.

(b) Valve dysfunction

The valves of the heart allow a non-return flow system and valve dysfunction, either stenosis, regurgitation or a combination of these, will decrease the efficiency of the heart as a pump and place a greater work load on the myocardium. Dysfunction of a heart valve may be due to congenital malformation, rheumatic fever, bacterial, viral or fungal infection, degenerative changes, collagen disease (e.g. Marfan's syndrome), or rarely due to direct or indirect trauma.

Valve dysfunction may be acute and severe, precipitating early heart failure in a previously healthy heart. It is more commonly a chronic malfunction present for many years before finally severe heart failure ensues. The myocardium adapts to the increased work load by hypertrophy, but finally failure occurs due to increasing deterioration of the valve function beyond the dynamic capabilities of the myocardium. Sometimes an additional factor is marked myocardial hypertrophy 'outgrowing' the coronary blood supply with detrimental relative ischaemia. Secondary myocardial damage was thought to be very significant but with the advent of heart valve replacement it has been shown that the valve dysfunction is by far the most important factor in the great majority of cases. The time of onset of failure is related to the severity of the valve dysfunction, and it is only when the cardiac output begins to become reduced that major myocardial damage occurs. It is from this point that myocardial damage becomes progressively significant. Once a heart valve is damaged it will subsequently show gradual progressive deterioration even if the precipitating cause is completely eradicated.

A patient already taking cardiac drugs who develops cardiac failure associated with valve disease needs correction of the valve dysfunction by operation before satisfactory control of the failure is possible. The high-grade postoperative care that is necessary in patients who have undergone heart operations has been one of the main stimuli in the development of the ICU.

(c) Generalised inadequate myocardial oxygenation

The heart requires an adequate oxygen supply for its metabolism. It has a high work load and its oxygen demand is so great that approximately 3–5 % of the cardiac output passes through the coronary circulation under basal conditions. Any condition that reduces the oxygen delivery, for example anaemia, low cardiac output and anoxia, will reduce the myocardial function.

Hypoxia is the common pathway in most cases of myocardial decompensation. Whatever the factors are that initiate the cardiovascular stress, the subsequent low cardiac output will cause inadequate myocardial oxygenation. Once significant myocardial hypoxia becomes established a vicious circle is set up which, unless broken, progresses to cardiac arrest (Fig. 2.2).

(d) Dysrhythmias

Sinus rhythm is the most efficient form of myocardial contraction. Any change from this rhythm is associated with a reduction in cardiac efficiency; for instance, atrial fibrillation reduces the cardiac output by approximately 30 % and ventricular fibrillation produces no effective cardiac output. Dysrhythmias may be precipitated by many causes including hypoxia, acidaemia, hypercapnia (page 93), hypokalaemia or hyperkalaemia, hyponatremia or hypernatremia, drug toxicity or operative trauma. On occasions the cause cannot be identified.

The treatment is related to the type of dysrhythmia and also to the cause if this is known. It is necessary to understand the normal electrocardiogram tracing before abnormal rhythms can be appreciated.

The normal electrocardiogram (ECG)

All muscle produces electrical activity during contraction and the electrocardiogram is a recording taken, by means of a galvanometer, of the electrical activity produced by cardiac muscle contraction.

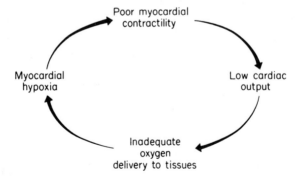

Fig. 2.2 The vicious circle in myocardial decompensation which leads to cardiac arrest

The electrocardiogram tracing is made on recording paper which has horizontal and vertical lines of which each fifth one is emphasised. The horizontal lines allow the deflection of the ECG to be measured, each line being 1 mm apart which represents 0.1 mV. The vertical lines show the time intervals and are similarly 1 mm apart each representing 0.04 seconds; each darker fifth line therefore represents 0.2 seconds (Fig. 2.3). The ECG displayed on an oscilloscope screen is set to sweep at either 25 mm/s or 50 mm/s. The faster speed is useful when subtle changes in complexes are suspected.

There are two basic types of recordings, bipolar and unipolar. In bipolar recordings two electrodes are put on the surface of the body at separate points and the differences in electrical potential produced by the contracting heart at the two points is measured. These are known as the *standard leads:*

standard lead I is between the left and right arms;
standard lead II is between the right arm and left leg;
standard lead III is between the left leg and left arm.

In unipolar recordings one of the two electrodes remains at zero potential and the other electrode is used to measure that electrical potential at its point of contact. The unipolar leads are:

aVL from the left arm;
aVR from the right arm;
aVF from the left leg.

The unipolar *chest* or *precordial leads* are designated V_1, V_2, V_3, V_4, V_5 and V_6. The position of these electrodes is shown in Fig. 2.4. While any of

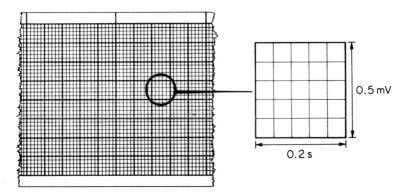

0.5 mV

0.2 s

Fig. 2.3 ECG recording paper. The horizontal lines spaced 1 mm apart show the amplitude; one centimetre corresponds to one millivolt. The vertical lines spaced 1 mm apart show the time interval, each small space representing 0.04 seconds when the paper is running at the normal speed of 25 mm/s. Subtle changes in the ECG may be more closely observed by using a faster speed of 50 mm/s.

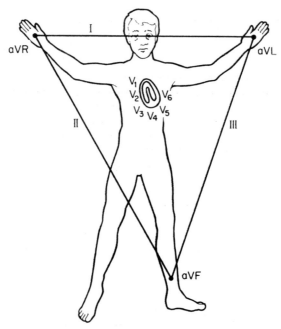

Fig. 2.4 Diagrammatic representation of the reference points of the basic ECG recordings. When using the CM5 configuration the left arm should be placed in the V_5 position (anterior axillary line, 5th intercostal space), the right arm lead should be placed over or slightly to the right of the manubrium sterni, and the indifferent lead may be placed on any convenient position

the standard limb leads (I, II, III, aVR, aVL, aVF) may be used for continuous monitoring, they have the disadvantage of having relatively low voltages and particularly of being poor indicators of myocardial ischaemia. The bipolar lead CM5 (Central Manubrium, and 5th interspace in the left anterior axillary line) is probably the best for routine monitoring in the ICU especially in patients with left ventricular disease (e.g. hypertension and ischaemic heart disease) and the cardiomyopathies. The CM5 lead is one of the best single leads, being able to detect ST segment changes in a higher proportion of patients than any other single lead.

Each normal sinus contraction of the heart produces on the ECG a series of deflections (Fig. 2.5). These are described as follows:

P wave. A first deflection of small amplitude corresponding to atrial contraction. Normally the P wave is less than 2.5 mm (0.25 mV) in amplitude and less than 0.1 s in duration. The normal P wave is upward in I and II and downward in aVR. There is then a latent period when there is no muscular contraction during conduction of the impulse from the atria to the ventricles (atrio-ventricular conduction).

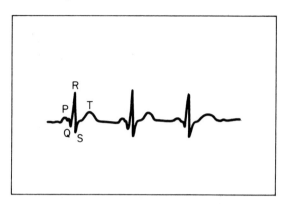

Fig. 2.5 The normal electrocardiogram, standard lead 1. Note the regularity of the cardiac cycle and the normal time relationships of the sinus complexes

P	atrial wave, less than 0.1 s
PR	atrio-ventricular conduction, 0.12–0.20 s
QRS	rapid ventricular depolarisation, usually 0.05–0.08 s
T	slow ventricular repolarisation wave

QRS waves. There follows a ventricular complex composed of rapid large deflections representing right and left ventricular contraction. The first deflection is downwards (Q wave), the second upward (R wave) and the third downward (S wave). These may be of varying amplitude. The complex can be normally up to 0.12 s in duration. It can have variable form but is normally upwards (R wave) in I and V_5 and downwards (S wave) in aVR and V_1.

T wave. The ventricular complex also has a T wave which is sometimes followed by a U wave. The latter is always small. The T wave corresponds to the disappearance of the stimulus in the ventricles and is generally accepted as representing an electrical repolarisation wave. Its maximum duration is 0.18–0.22 s. It is usually upwards except in aVR when it is normally downwards.

PR interval. This is the time interval between the beginning of the P wave and the beginning of the R wave and represents the atrio-ventricular conduction time. It has a normal duration of 0.12–0.20 s.

The common dysrhythmias

(i) Ventricular fibrillation. This is usually a terminal dysrhythmia unless immediately treated. The heart is completely non-functional owing to chaotic, patchy, totally disorganised myocardial fibrillary contraction. The ECG is characterised by bizarre irregular deflections (Fig. 2.6).

(ii) Ventricular asystole. This is the other form of terminal dys-rhythmia, in which the ventricles are at a complete standstill. Usually

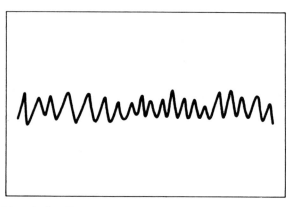

Fig. 2.6 Ventricular fibrillation. Note the rapid bizarre irregular deflections

there are no other electrocardiographic deflections (or only a very few low amplitude wide complexes), the ECG being essentially a flat trace. This type of dysrhythmia is much more common in children than in adults and is often preceded by a period of bradycardia. Conversely it is uncommon for children to exhibit ventricular fibrillation as a terminal dysrhythmia. Severe myocardial anoxia is the usual feature in asystole. It is possible for an intravenous injection of potassium to cause asystolic arrest if the injection is given too rapidly.

These two dysrhythmias produce complete circulatory arrest and immediate treatment is required.

Management of cardiac arrest

The immediate priorities to maintain life are restoration of the circulation by closed chest massage and maintenance of adequate ventilation.

Satisfactory massage requires the patient to be lying on a firm base and all intensive care beds should have a solid board under the mattress to satisfy this requirement. If there is no firm support the patient should be rapidly transferred to the floor. The resuscitator's hands should be crossed and placed on top of each other, palm down, on to the lower half of the sternum centred a little to the left (Fig. 2.7). Firm intermittent pressure is applied to the heart by downward compression of the chest wall, at a rate of approximately 80–100 per minute and the compression phase should be rapid to gain as much acceleration of blood flow as possible. It is easiest to satisfy these requirements by a straight arm action with most of the movement and force coming from bending at the waist. Adequate massage by this method can be continued by the same person for long periods of time without exhaustion. Someone should ensure that the massage is maintaining an adequate circulation by checking that the patient's pupils remain non-dilated and that each massage produces a palpable femoral pulse.

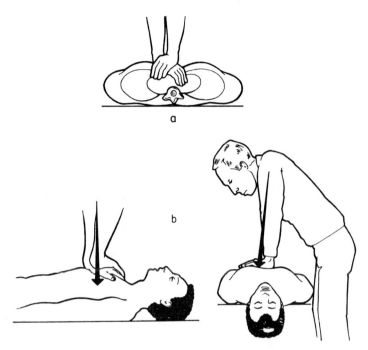

Fig. 2.7 Closed chest cardiac massage; (a) the sternum is compressed by the heels of crossed palms 80–100 times per minute; (b) the full weight of the body is applied by a straight arm, waist bending movement

In larger children adequate cardiac massage is gained by using only one hand and this reduces the chance of producing damage to the chest wall and contained organs. In infants the site of compression should be the mid-sternum as the heart lies relatively higher in the chest. In young children it is relatively easy to rupture the liver and if the thorax can be grasped in the hand adequate massage can be gained by compressing the sternum with the thumb. The optimal compression frequency is of the order of 100 per minute with lung inflation every 5 cycles (20:1 ratio).

The second most important requirement to restoring circulation is to ensure adequate ventilation. The patient will in almost all cases be unconscious and an endotracheal tube should be inserted and positive pressure respiration with 100 % oxygen maintained by an anaesthetic bag. Mouth to mouth respiration should not be necessary as tracheal intubation should always be immediately available in an ICU. Time should not however be wasted in attempting a difficult intubation. The lungs can be satisfactorily inflated by a face mask and self-filling bag (e.g. Laerdal or Ambu bag). The instruction of junior hospital staff and intensive care nurses in the technique of tracheal intubation is as important as training in cardiac massage and defibrillation. Very rarely, a patient will regain consciousness during cardiac massage, and in this case it may be necessary to paralyse and sedate the patient (see page 76).

The third most important requirement is to ensure that there is free access for intravenous injections. If an intravenous catheter is not already *in situ*, a major vein catheterisation (i.e. subclavian or internal jugular) can be easily and rapidly performed. To control the tendency to acidosis, which always occurs owing to the fact that the maximum rate of circulation during massage is only 35% of normal, an immediate intravenous injection of 100 ml of 8.4% sodium bicarbonate (100 mmol $NaHCO_3$) should be given to adults unless there has been no delay in recognition of the arrest in a previously well oxygenated and perfused patient. A proportional volume equivalent to 1 mmol $NaHCO_3$ per kilogram should be given to children. If the arrest persists, necessitating continued cardiac massage, further doses of half the initial volume of $NaHCO_3$ should be given every 10 minutes. This regime should control the acid-base balance satisfactorily during the period of cardiac massage but pH check measurements should be performed on samples of arterial blood if possible. Uncorrected acidaemia may be the cause of failure of defibrillation.

If ventricular fibrillation is present an external direct current (DC) defibrillation shock of 160–200 joules should be given as soon as possible. It is very important that the external electrodes are well smeared with electrode jelly right out to their edges to avoid skin burns and ensure maximal electrical contact. The electrodes should be placed so that the defibrillation impulse is directed across the heart. One electrode should be placed firmly to the right of the mid-sternum, the second should be placed over the presumed or known level of the cardiac apex between the anterior and mid-axillary lines of the left chest (Fig. 2.8). It is safer if each electrode is held by a different person to remove all possibility of the apparatus shorting across a medical attendant holding both electrodes. If a defibrillator is immediately to hand when ventricular fibrillation occurs, this should be used at once instead of cardiac massage and ventilation. If immediate electroconversion is obtained cardiac massage is avoided. This should be attempted only if the defibrillator is immediately available and the counter-shock can be given without delay.

If ventricular asystole is present it is necessary to regain myocardial tone before a synchronous contraction can be obtained. The treatment of asystole or resistant ventricular fibrillation is essentially the same. While the cardiac massage is continued intravenous injection of cardiotonic drugs are given—0.01 mg isoprenaline or 0.1 mg adrenaline, and 10 ml of 10% calcium gluconate.*

---

* In some hospitals calcium chloride is used instead; care is needed because there are three different preparations of calcium chloride available—the hydrate, the dihydrate and the hexahydrate salts. The amount of calcium varies according to the formulation (page 221).

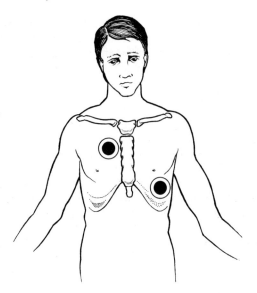

Fig. 2.8 Diagram illustrating the position of placement of external defibrillator electrodes

At the same time any acidosis is corrected by intravenous sodium bicarbonate and satisfactory ventilation is maintained. Any other detrimental factors such as hypovolaemia must be corrected as far as possible before a further defibrillation is attempted. Persistent attempts at defibrillation in the presence of hypoxia are harmful. The aim should be to get as good cardiac massage as possible with good oxygenation before defibrillation is attempted.

If asystole persists despite all treatment, recovery is impossible and it must be assumed that there is a major detrimental factor that cannot be relieved. Cardiac massage for longer than 30 minutes under these conditions is not indicated and death should be accepted. Attempts to stimulate myocardial contraction in asystolic arrest by electrical pacing are never successful as the persisting asystole is due to underlying severe myocardial anoxia which negates any form of contraction. It is important to exclude certain drugs as causative agents (e.g. the very lipophilic local anaesthetic bupivacaine, when asystole may persist for as long as 75 minutes).

If ventricular fibrillation is resistant to electroconversion every effort should be made to ensure all apsects of the cardiac massage are satisfactory and are continued for a prolonged time to gain as good a myocardial perfusion as possible. A 5–10 minute period of uninterrupted massage should be given before repeating the cardiotonic drugs and re-attempting defibrillation. Ventricular fibrillation persisting despite all treatment can be converted to asystole by rapid intravenous injection of 40 mmol potassium chloride. The massage is continued during the subsequent asystolic period and as the effect wears off after 3—5 minutes, spontaneous synchronised contractions may commence. If ventricular fibrillation redevelops a DC countershock may then be successful. It is usual to continue cardiac massage for much longer periods in resistant ventricular fibrillation than in persistent asystole as the very presence of myocardial activity indicates some degree of myocardial perfusion with the implied potential of regaining synchronised contractions. If the fibrillation persists despite all efforts for 45—60 minutes, death should be accepted. If defibrillation is successful but fibrillation repeatedly reasserts itself, intermittent massage may be indicated for much longer periods and drugs to reduce cardiac excitability may be indicated. In these cases ventricular pacing may suppress the dysrhythmic tendency. Causes of fixed dilated pupils such as quinine overdosage and the use of inotropes must be remembered. There are many recorded instances of cardiac postoperative cases and postinfarction patients walking out of hospital after many episodes of ventricular fibrillation.

(iii) Ventricular tachycardia. This is a rapid ventricular rhythm generally faster than 140 per minute. The rate may be regular or may fluctuate slightly over short periods of time. The ventricular origin of the contraction is indicated by the altered form of the QRS complex on the ECG which is widespread, large and often hooked (Fig. 2.9). This rhythm usually indicates myocardial anoxia, which may be made worse, and the T waves are inverted. Ventricular tachycardia may be precipitated by overdosage of drugs such as adrenaline, isoprenaline and digoxin. The rhythm is very inefficient and will precipitate or aggravate heart failure.

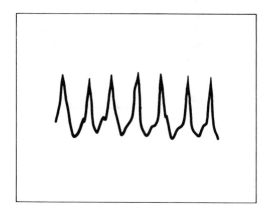

Fig. 2.9 Ventricular tachycardia. The close relationship between ventricular tachycardia and ventricular extrasystoles is seen. Each beat in the paroxysm resembles a ventricular extrasystole having a widespread excursion with inverted T wave

Ventricular tachycardia is a frequent precursor of ventricular fibrillation and it is imperative that active treatment is initiated.

Direct current (DC) counter-shock is the preferred method of treatment, although intravenous lignocaine or procaine amide may be used. An ultrashort-acting barbiturate anaesthetic such as methohexitone is suitable for this purpose and ventilation and intubation should be unnecessary. If the patient is adequately sedated the counter-shock can be given without an anaesthetic. At the same time any acidosis or hypoxia should be corrected.

(iv) Ventricular extrasystole. This is an extra beat of the heart with the excitatory focus in the ventricular muscles as in ventricular tachycardia; the ECGs are similar (Fig. 2.10). Each premature beat is followed by a pause which is usually compensatory; that is, the time from the normal beat preceding to that following the extrasystole is exactly equal to the time between three normal beats. Ventricular tachycardia is a continuous run of ventricular extrasystoles. The occurrence of ventricular extrasystoles usually indicates myocardial anoxia and is a common dysrhythmia following myocardial infarction. If the precipitating cause increases there is an increasing rate of extrasystoles. This pattern is a very common precursor to ventricular tachycardia or fibrillation. The emergence of ventricular extrasystoles indicates an unsatisfactory state of affairs and it is important to check that the cardiac output is maintained, arterial oxygenation is satisfactory and an acid-base imbalance has not developed. In addition, intracellular hypokalaemia is a precipitating cause of ventricular instability and the intravenous injection of 10–20 mmol of potassium chloride will often dramatically reduce the incidence of ventricular dysrhythmias. This procedure is perfectly safe if it is ensured that the serum potassium level is not above normal and if the injection is made over several minutes into a peripheral vein.

If subsequently there is a continuing incidence of extrasystoles an intravenous infusion of lignocaine should be instituted which will depress the myocardial excitability and abolish or reduce the incidence of the

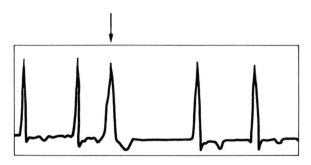

Fig. 2.10 Ventricular extrasystole. An isolated ventricular extrasystole with post-extrasystolic ischaemia showing in addition a compensatory pause

dysrhythmia. A maximal rate of 250 mg of lignocaine per hour should be observed.

Practolol is a useful anti-dysrhythmic drug for suppressing ventricular ectopic activity. It is not necessary to produce beta-adrenergic blockade in order to achieve the effect and small intravenous doses of about 1–5 mg are usually adequate. Repeated doses can be given every 15 minutes to a maximum dose of 20 mg. Intravenous doses larger than this can produce severe myocardial depression.

Bigeminal ventricular extrasystole. This is a coupled rhythm when the extrasystole occurs after each sinus contraction (Fig. 2.11). It is classically associated with digoxin toxicity. It should be noted that intracellular hypokalaemia renders the myocardium more sensitive to digoxin and coupling may occur under these conditions even if the digoxin level is below the 'toxicity' level. The effects of digoxin toxicity can be relieved or ameliorated by intravenous injection of potassium or practolol as previously described. Potassium injections should not be given to patients in renal failure.

Pacing the heart

In open heart operations it is usual practice to insert epicardial pacemaker electrodes before closing the chest. If required, these wires allow immediate pacemaker control of the heart during the postoperative period. The electrode wires are gently pulled out on the seventh postoperative day when the patient is convalescent. In other conditions requiring intensive care of the cardiovascular system when the chest has not been open, there should always be an endocardial co-axial electrode catheter immediately available. If the need arises this catheter can be quickly inserted into the right side of the heart via a peripheral vein in the same way as a central venous catheter. X-ray control is not necessary in urgent cases as blind insertion of an electrode catheter will afford reasonable pacemaker control. Under these conditions the catheter tip may not be optimally placed and a high voltage may be necessary to gain control of heart contraction. This will only be satisfactory to maintain pacing for a short period. Accurate placing of the electrode catheter by X-ray screening can be performed later with no urgency.

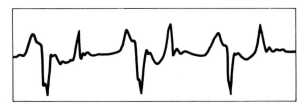

Fig. 2.11 Bigeminal ventricular extrasystoles. These produce a coupled rhythm, the extrasystole occurring after each sinus contraction

External pacemaker electrodes are available which can be applied to the chest wall but this requires a high energy system and is very painful.

Atrial pacing produces a more efficient synchronised contraction than ventricular pacing and should be used whenever possible. Long term stable atrial pacing by means of an endocardial catheter is difficult to obtain owing to the difficulty of impacting the tip of the catheter. Atrial pacing is of course impossible in a condition of total heart block when only ventricular pacing can be used.

Pacemaker machines may give only a regular or fixed rate impulse or, better, include demand pacing circuits. The latter will allow a stimulus only if the intrinsic heart rate slows below a rate which can be selected. This ensures that the pacemaker activity does not continue if and when a satisfactory intrinsic rhythm is regained. In addition, the demand system ensures that a pacemaker stimulus does not reach the heart during the sensitive period at the beginning of the T wave when ventricular fibrillation can be precipitated. This risk is, however, much less than was originally thought.

Indications for pacemaker control of the heart
1 Any resistant bradycardic condition when the cardiac output is unsatisfactory:
   (*a*) severe sinus bradycardia which will not respond to atropine or isoprenaline
   (*b*) nodal bradycardia (junctional bradycardia)
   (*c*) heart block
2 Persisting ventricular dysrhythmias which may be controlled by atrial pacing at a higher initial rate than the existing intrinsic rhythm.

Whenever possible atrial pacing is preferred to ventricular pacing except in total heart block.

(v) Nodal rhythm (junctional rhythm). This occurs when the sino-atrial node becomes suppressed; the atrio-ventricular node takes over, giving rise to a nodal rhythm. It may give rise to scattered nodal extrasystoles or to paroxysmal nodal tachycardia or less commonly bradycardia. These can be precipitated by vagotonic reflexes, digoxin, quinidine or in disease conditions where there is myocarditis or in myocardial stress, e.g. infarction. It can occasionally be seen in normal individuals. In this rhythm the atrial activation, indicated by the P wave in the ECG, is abnormally sited either before, during or after the activation of the ventricle. There are, therefore, three types of nodal rhythm: upper, average and lower (Fig. 2.12).

Nodal rhythm is less malignant than the ventricular dysrhythmias and can maintain an acceptable circulation for many hours. It is virtually never a stable rhythm and will eventually deteriorate to a ventricular rhythm or improve to an atrial rhythm. In conditions of low cardiac output the heart often deteriorates into a nodal rhythm but if the cardiac

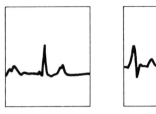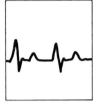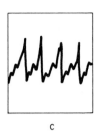

a   b   c

Fig. 2.12 (a) Upper nodal rhythm with the P wave immediately before the QRS; (b) average nodal rhythm when the P waves are not visible, being lost within the ventricular QRS complex; (c) low nodal rhythm with a typically negative P wave following the ventricular complex

output can be improved normal rhythm will usually re-establish itself spontaneously. Active treatment in addition to that aimed at increasing the cardiac output includes electroconversion, intravenous practolol and atrial pacing. When the cardiac output is low in association with a nodal bradycardia, which is resistant to isoprenaline infusion, it is necessary to pace the heart at a faster rate. If atrial pacing cannot be obtained then ventricular pacing should be established.

Both ventricular and nodal dysrhythmias may be precipitated by digoxin especially if there is coexistent hypokalaemia. In general digoxin is not indicated in these dysrhythmias and if the patient is already taking this drug it should be stopped. At the same time if the serum potassium level is not above normal, potassium chloride should be given intravenously at the rate of 80–120 mmol per 24 hours in the adult.

The tendency to nodal rhythms may be reduced or suppressed by intravenous lignocaine as described in ventricular dysrhythmias. 200 mg of phenytoin given intravenously may also be effective. These drugs, however, are more effective in controlling ventricular dysrhythmias.

(vi) Atrial flutter and fibrillation. In this condition the atria cease to contract properly with very rapid atrial stimuli resulting in disorganised activity of the atrial myocardium. This rhythm is associated with a 30 % reduction in the cardiac output. In *flutter* the atrial waves occur at the rate of 200–400 per minute. The atrio-ventricular node cannot respond to every atrial stimulus and will respond only to every second or third stimulus producing a 2:1 or 3:1 block. This produces a ventricular rate of approximately 100–200 per minute which is regular. In *atrial fibrillation* the atrial stimuli are very numerous at 400–700 per minute and the ventricles respond in a totally irregular tachycardia (Fig. 2.13).

The onset of these atrial dysrhythmias usually indicates that one or both atria are under stress and that there is raised atrial pressure. This is commonly seen in mitral stenosis and in any cause of right or left ventricular failure in older adults. An untreated atrial dysrhythmia

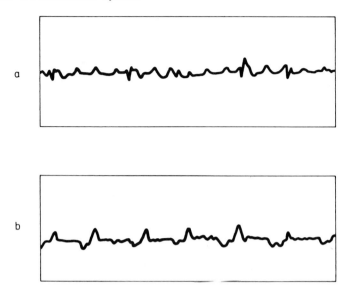

Fig. 2.13 (a) Atrial flutter with a varying 2:1 and 4:1 block; (b) atrial fibrillation with a slow but totally irregular ventricular rate in a digitalised patient

always causes a reduction in cardiac efficiency and often precipitates cardiac failure.

The treatment of both these dysrhythmias is similar. Electroconversion by DC counter-shock, if successful, has the advantage of restoring normal rhythm. Digitalisation in atrial fibrillation will slow the ventricular response and narrow the pulse deficit, making the heart action more efficient. In atrial flutter, digitalisation has the possible disadvantage of increasing the ventricular rate by reducing the atrial rate but at the same time reducing the degree of block. Treatment with practolol will also slow the ventricular response and is probably the drug of choice in atrial flutter. In conditions of severe cardiac failure atrial fibrillation may persistently fail to respond to counter-shock and may also fail to become controlled despite full digitalisation. A very high ventricular rate may persist with a large pulse deficit. It is incorrect to administer more digoxin with its dangers of toxicity. It is becoming increasingly possible to measure digoxin blood levels and this will confirm that there is adequate digitalisation. The lack of control of the atrial fibrillation is related to underlying unsatisfactory myocardial factors which are not understood but the administration of practolol will usually improve the degree of control.

(vii) Heart block. Atrio-ventricular block results from an arrest or slowing of the stimulus from the atria to the ventricles. There are three types of block:

First degree block. Conduction across from the atria to the ventricles is slowed. This is shown in the ECG by an increased PR interval beyond the upper normal of 0.2 seconds (Fig. 2.14).

Second degree block. This is usually a 2:1 block when only alternate P waves are followed by a QRS complex, the ventricles beating at half the atrial rate (i.e. about 40 per minute) (Fig. 2.15). Occasionally the Wenckebach phenomenon is seen where the PR interval steadily lengthens until the P wave is not followed by a ventricular response. This cycle continually repeats itself (Fig. 2.16).

Complete atrio-ventricular block. This occurs when there is complete dissociation between the atrial and ventricular activity. The P waves are

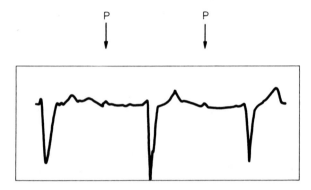

Fig. 2.14 First degree heart block. The conduction in the bundle of His is slow but not interupted. It shows itself as an abnormally long PR interval, 0.56 s in this tracing

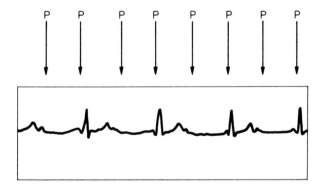

Fig. 2.15 Second degree heart block, 2:1 type. Every other P wave is followed by a QRS (ventricular complex)

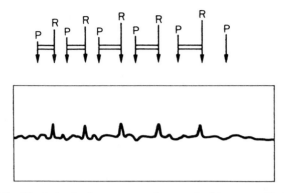

Fig. 2.16 The Wenkebach phenomenon characterised by a steadily lengthening PR interval until the P wave occurs without a ventricular response. The cycle is then repeated

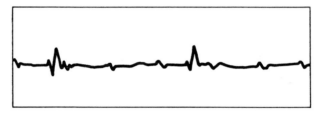

Fig. 2.17 Complete heart block with the complete dissociation between the atria (P waves) and the ventricles (QRS complex)

regular at a rate of 60–80 per minute. The ventricular complexes are variably deformed and are regular, slower and completely unrelated to the P waves (Fig. 2.17).

The haemodynamic effect of first degree heart block is not important and no specific therapy is necessary. In total and sometimes second degree heart block the slow ventricular rate produces a significantly low cardiac output. In addition Stokes-Adams attacks may occur. These are brief periods of unconsciousness due to circulatory standstill related to brief periods of ventricular arrest or fibrillation. Urgent treatment is required and if spontaneous contractions do not rapidly return death occurs.

The injection of a chronotropic drug such as isoprenaline will speed the ventricular rate to a small extent and may reduce the degree of block if the precipitating cause is poor myocardial oxygenation due to poor coronary flow, rather than myocardial damage. In most cases, heart block is persistent enough to demand ventricular pacing and this is the treatment of choice. If the block is persistent it is very dangerous to depend on an isoprenaline drip to maintain an acceptable heart rate. Rapid tolerance to isoprenaline can develop in these cases with early return to a low cardiac output and recurrence of Stokes-Adams attacks.

The commonest causes of heart block are ischaemia following myocardial infarction, trauma in cardiac surgery, hypoxia in low cardiac output states, and 'idiopathic' when heart block suddenly occurs in an otherwise apparently healthy person. The latter appears to be related to local degeneration in the conducting tissue of the heart.

If heart block presents in the ICU pacemaker control must always be established with correction of the low cardiac output as soon as possible.

ECG abnormalities related to metabolism, drugs and the endocrine system. The ECG changes described below are characteristic but are of very little value in diagnosis as there is marked individual variation:

Hypokalaemia. This leads to an increase in the QT interval with a flattened T wave which may become absent or biphasic and is associated with a second U wave.

Hyperkalaemia and hypercalcaemia. The ECG shows high peaked narrow T waves and there is a short QT interval which can proceed to asystole.

Hypothyroidism. This condition is characterised by sinus bradycardia with low voltage complexes, flattened or negative T waves. The same type of tracing can be obtained in constrictive pericarditis.

Hyperthyroidism. There is characteristically an unstable tachycardia with large T waves which is frequently associated with paroxysmal or sustained atrial fibrillation.

Cardiac glycosides, e.g. digoxin. As digitalisation is obtained there is shortening of the QT interval, dipping of the ST interval and rounding of the T wave to a characteristic dome shape. Overdosage with digoxin produces increasing delay in conduction across the bundle of His and increasing ventricular instability. Classically, bigeminal ventricular extrasystoles develop (see page 26). Increasing toxicity leads to multiple ventricular extrasystoles which can progress to ventricular tachycardia and finally fibrillation. Warning bigeminal ventricular extrasystoles do not always develop and the toxicity may suddenly declare itself by gross ventricular instability.

(e)   Tamponade and constriction of the heart

If the heart is enclosed and compressed by blood or fluid in the pericardial cavity or is gripped by pericardial fibrosis, its contractions are physically restricted and the cardiac output will drop. Tamponade is a relatively rare cause of acute cardiovascular failure. It is seen occasionally after heart operations due to haemorrhage into an inadequately draining pericardial space and very rarely in other conditions of intrapericardial haemorrhage or acute effusions, e.g. uraemia, leukaemia, sharp penetrating wounds, pericardial malignant secondary deposits and certain viral infections. Constrictive pericarditis is a chronic form of tamponade due to the constricting fibrosis of the pericardium which may follow tuberculous or viral pericarditis.

In both cases there is a high CVP associated with a low cardiac output. Other clinical features of tamponade are an increasing heart silhouette on serial X-rays and a feeble pulse becoming weaker on inspiration (pulsus paradoxus). The heart sounds are said to become muffled and the cardiac apex becomes difficult or impossible to locate. These signs are by no means always present and are often inconclusive.

The diagnosis can nearly always be established by the isoprenaline test. Administration of isoprenaline in cases of tamponade or constriction produces the usual response of tachycardia and an initial dip in the systemic blood pressure as in any other form of cardiovascular failure. The virtually pathognomic sign is a rise in the CVP whereas in all other forms of failure the CVP falls. If this test is positive when tamponade is suspected, pericardial aspiration is obligatory. This is performed by careful exploration of the pericardial cavity in the area of the cardiac apex either by inserting an aspiration needle directly through the chest wall, or inserting it from below upwards deep to the xiphisternum. If the patient is on anticoagulants these must be antagonised.

Tamponade due to haemopericardium is most common in postoperative cardiac surgical patients, in which case the chest is re-opened as a matter of urgency. Complete evacuation of the blood is a simple matter and a direct search can be made for the bleeding point. If pericardial haemorrhage continues in non-surgical cases it is also necessary to operatively expose the pericardial cavity to gain control of the bleeding. In cases of pericardial effusion causing cardiac tamponade it is possible to insert a fine catheter to drain the pericardial space. This is inserted as for vein catheterisation by careful puncture of the pericardium from under the xiphisternum.

(f) Electrolyte imbalance

Imbalance of electrolytes can depress myocardial contractility or increase its instability. There are many possible causes of electrolyte imbalance but the common final effect is the same. The concentrations of the intracellular electrolytes and organic substances differ considerably from those of the extracellular fluids (Fig. 2.18). The integrity of the cell membrane maintains this difference and its function in turn depends on normally functioning enzymic mechanisms located on the cell mitochondria. If the cell becomes anoxic or there is a build up of toxins or toxic chemicals the enzyme systems become slowed, inhibited or destroyed and the cell

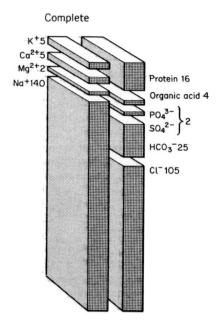

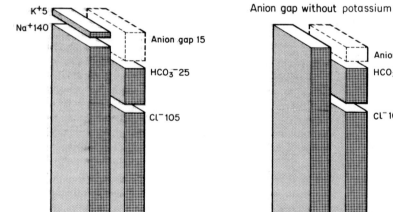

Anion gap = (Na⁺ + K⁺) − (Cl⁻ + HCO₃⁻)   Anion gap = Na⁺ − (Cl⁻ + HCO₃⁻)

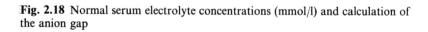

Fig. 2.18 Normal serum electrolyte concentrations (mmol/l) and calculation of the anion gap

membrane function progressively fails. As a result, the cell permeability increases and there is a tendency for equalisation of electrolyte concentrations between the cell and the interstitial fluid. Potassium moves out of the cell and sodium moves in. There is also water movement into the cell and this results in increasing intracellular oedema. These changes are associated with mitochondrial swelling and fragmentation; at first the process is reversible but with increasing cell damage it becomes irreversible and progresses to cell death.

In conditions of cardiovascular stress it is important to control electrolyte homeostasis as far as possible. Myocardial stability depends on the intracellular electrolyte concentrations and also on the concentration gradient across the cell wall. The most common abnormality is intracellular hypokalaemia. The kidneys excrete the increased potassium liberated from the cells and the serum potassium level remains within normal range (3.5–5.6 mmol/l). In this way all but gross potassium deficiency is usually concealed unless renal failure co-exists. The intracellular deficiency increases the myocardial irritability, increasing the tendency to ventricular rhythmias and fibrillation. In addition the myocardium is rendered more sensitive to digoxin.

A patient in cardiovascular failure virtually always has a low intracellular potassium and if on diuretics, hypokalaemia is a certainty. Even the usual administration of potassium supplements with diuretics only partially controls the potassium depletion. The sodium moves in the opposite direction into the cells and as a result the intracellular sodium is high and the extracellular sodium tends to be low, this being reflected by a relatively low serum sodium (normal range 135–150 mmol/l). At the same time the water which accompanies the sodium movement renders the cells overhydrated. This partially explains why the serum sodium progressively drops in cases of increasing heart failure. It is important to replace any sodium or potassium losses whether the loss is external (in the urine, sweat or faeces) or internal (into the cells or body cavities).

A patient in severe cardiac failure on heavy diuretic drive and in low cardiac output often develops a low serum sodium concentration due to the above mechanism. In this circumstance although there may be a high intracellular sodium and a normal or high total body sodium, the response to the diuretic may cease owing to the low serum sodium, and the patient becomes oliguric with progressive deterioration and oedema. A satisfactory diuresis will only be gained in these cases if intravenous saline is given to supply salt to the stressed kidneys. The renal excretion of water is always associated with a small but obligatory loss of salt and this also applies in kidneys which are poorly perfused due to a low cardiac output.

Intravenous injections of ionic calcium stimulate the heart to contract more forcibly and a low serum ionic calcium can be associated with weakened myocardial contractions. The serum level of calcium (normal range 2.2–2.5 mol/l blood) is however very accurately controlled and the level drops below normal only in a very few diseases, such as

parathyroid tetany, steatorrhoea and other forms of protracted diarrhoea. In conditions of massive haemorrhage 5–10 ml of 10 % calcium
gluconate may be given with every unit of transfused bank blood. This is
to counteract the calcium binding effect of the citrate in the bank blood
which renders the calcium physiologically inactive. However, the metabolic control of the serum calcium level is so powerful that calcium
injections are only important when virtual total blood volume replacement occurs. The need for calcium therapy of this kind is greatly reduced
by avoiding the transfusion of cold blood.

It has been shown that imbalance of other electrolytes such as
magnesium may also play a part in myocardial dysfunction.
Unfortunately, intracellular electrolyte determinations are not routinely
available in hospital practice and the administration of electrolytes must
be decided upon from indirect information, such as 24-hourly urine
excretions and serum levels coupled with clinical experience. The facility
of intracellular electrolyte estimations is one of the most pressing
requirements in clinical work today.

(g)   Acid-base imbalance

Acidity is produced by free hydrogen ions in solution. The acidity of a
solution is measured by the hydrogen ion concentration and expressed as
the pH, the lower the pH the more acid is the solution (see page 62). The
control of the acid-base balance is by the kidneys, which can excrete or
retain acids as required, by the respiratory system which can eliminate
carbonic acid in the form of carbon dioxide and water, and by the buffers
in the blood. Buffers are substances that can accept or donate hydrogen
ions and when present in a solution tend to hold the free hydrogen ion
concentration, and therefore the pH, at a fixed level, even if acids or
alkalis are added to the solution. The important buffering substances in
the blood are bicarbonate and haemoglobin. The buffering power of the
body is therefore decreased in anaemia.

Metabolic acid-base disturbances are caused by the accumulation or
loss of either acid or base from sources other than carbon dioxide. Such
disturbances will promote either acidosis or alkalosis respectively. The
blood pH may not reveal these disturbances until there is failure of the
buffer systems and the hydrogen ion concentration becomes abnormal,
i.e. acidaemia or alkalaemia develops, which is a serious situation.

Normal values of hydrogen ion concentration in arterial blood are pH
7.36–7.44. The limits of blood hydrogen ion concentration generally
compatible with survival are pH 6.8–7.7. The normal values for arterial
P_{CO_2} at 37°C are 36–44 mmHg (4.80–5.87 kPa) and the plasma bicarbonate concentrate is about 24 mmol/l. The total carbon dioxide
concentration in the blood is about 25.2 mmol/l; the small difference
between this value and the plasma bicarbonate represents the small
amount of CO_2 physically carried in the plasma. Actual bicarbonate

concentrations are calculated from measured pH and P_{CO_2} values of whole blood samples introduced into electrode systems.

Terminology

Acidaemia is an abnormal state of blood in which the pH is too low.

Alkalaemia is an abnormal state of blood in which the pH is too high.

Respiratory acidosis (hypercapnia) is an abnormal process in which there is a primary decrease in the rate of alveolar ventilation relative to the rate of CO_2 production. A P_{CO_2} above normal limits describes an abnormal state of blood but this situation can either be a primary or a compensatory physiological process.

Respiratory alkalosis is an abnormal process in which there is a primary increase in the rate of alveolar ventilation relative to the rate of CO_2 production.

Metabolic acidosis is an abnormal physiological process in the body characterised by the primary gain of strong acid (e.g. lactic acid, the products of anaerobic metabolism) or the primary loss of bicarbonate from the extracellular fluid (e.g. small bowel fistulae).

Metabolic alkalosis is an abnormal physiological process characterised by the primary gain of strong base (e.g. overdosage by sodium bicarbonate) or by the primary loss of strong acid (e.g. hydrochloric acid lost in gastric aspirate, or vomiting) from the extracellular fluid.
The normal range of actual bicarbonate concentration is 22–26 mmol/l, and standard bicarbonate is a measure of the bicarbonate concentration under standard conditions (i.e. the plasma of fully oxygenated blood at a P_{CO_2} of 40 mmHg or 5.32 kPa at 37°C); normal values are 22–26 mmol/l.

Base excess BE (or deficit) represents the amount of strong acid (or base) to return the pH to 7.4 when the P_{CO_2} is 40 mmHg or 5.32 kPa at 37°C. The normal range of BE is 0 ± 2.5 mmol/l. Base excess can be computed from graphs, nomograms or the calculator unit of automatic blood gas analysers when pH or P_{CO_2} determinations have been made.

Controlling acid-base balance is very important in ICU patients. Low cardiac output results in increasing anaerobic cellular metabolism and increasing build-up of acids such as lactic acid; the result is a metabolic acidosis and a base deficit develops. A base deficit of more than 3 mmol/l may be corrected by multiplying this deficit by a third of the patient's weight in kilograms and giving this amount of bicarbonate (e.g. a base deficit of 6 mmol/l in a 70 kg patient would require 140 mmol of sodium bicarbonate). It is usual, however, to replace only about half this amount and then to repeat the acid-base analysis after an hour, giving more therapy if necessary. Bicarbonate therapy has the disadvantage that a largely unwanted sodium load is given and attention must be directed towards treating the cause of the acidosis (e.g. hypovolaemia, low cardiac output).

Arterial pH measurements indicate only the extracellular hydrogen ion concentration and do not show what is happening within the tissue cells; intracellular pH is always lower than extracellular pH. An arterial pH may show an alkalosis at the same time as an intracellular acidosis. This is occasionally seen in severe diabetic acidosis and some postoperative conditions. Although the blood is alkalotic the urine is acidotic and contains high amounts of potassium. Hypokalaemia will develop unless added potassium is given. The mechanism of intracellular acidosis in conjunction with extracellular alkalosis is not understood but is of serious importance. During the recovery stage the blood reverts to an acidotic state. The existence of a metabolic alkalosis in conditions of primary cardiovascular stress is always a bad sign and can only be concealing an intracellular acidosis. It is difficult to conceive of a low cardiac output being associated with anything other than a tissue acidosis except in the rare case of acute poisoning by alkali.

Humoral imbalance

With respect to the failing cardiovascular system a secondary failure of humoral factors is uncommon. In severe unresponsive cardiac failure sometimes hydrocortisone is injected, often in very large doses, in the vague hope that by augmenting the natural steroids there will be an improvement. This attitude became established because of the impressive, almost magical, properties of corticosteroids when they first became available, coupled with the clinical observation that intravenous administration of very large doses of hydrocortisone (2–3 g) produced an improvement in the peripheral perfusion of shocked patients. Subsequent investigations have shown that very high steroid levels have a separate direct peripheral vasodilator effect. Today, if a vasodilator effect is desired, it is usual to use more specific drugs such as phentolamine (Rogitine), sodium nitroprusside (Nipride), isosorbide, and glyceryl trinitrate BP or nitroglycerin USP (Tridil).

It is possible for a primary humoral imbalance to precipitate cardiovascular failure. Table 2.1 lists some specific endocrine diseases and their associated effects on the cardiovascular system. The treatment of any cardiovascular failure in these cases is the same as in any other cause. The specific treatment of the humoral disorder is equally important.

Table 2.1   Some effects of endocrine diseases on the cardiovascular system

Endocrine disease	Cardiovascular effects
Acromegaly	Cardiac enlargement Cardiomyopathy Congestive cardiac failure
Cushing's syndrome Adreno-cortical syndrome	Purpura Hypertension Congestive cardiac failure
Hyperthyroidism	Tachycardia Cardiac dysrhythmias especially atrial fibrillation Congestive cardiac failure
Hypothyroidism Pituitary myxoedema	Congestive cardiac failure Anaemia
Hypoparathyroidism	Congestive cardiac failure
Adreno-cortical insufficiency (Addison's Disease)	Purpura Cyanosis Severe hypotension Peripheral vascular failure
Phaeochromocytoma	Tachycardia Paroxysmal or sustained severe hypertension Congestive cardiac failure

Obstructed circulation—pulmonary embolus

When a thrombus embolises from a peripheral vein, through the right heart, into the pulmonary vascular tree the effect depends on the size of the embolus. If the pulmonary circulation is significantly obstructed by the embolus then right ventricular failure ensues and the patient requires intensive care.

The classical signs of pulmonary embolus are said to include sudden onset of breathlessness often with syncope or near syncope, tachycardia, hypotension, raised CVP, a third heart sound and pleuritic chest pain sometimes with haemoptysis. Only the pleuritic chest pain, haemoptysis and right ventricular failure are directly related to the obstructed pulmonary circulation, the other signs being non-specific and related to low cardiac output. The ECG is very important in respect to the diagnosis. The condition most likely to be confused with pulmonary embolus is myocardial infarction. The onset of the classical ECG changes in myocardial infarction may be delayed for up to 48 hours, but when there is serious obstruction to the pulmonary circulation from pulmonary embolus the classical ECG changes of acute right ventricular strain develop very quickly. The ECG changes are described as S_I, Q_{III}, T_{III}, there being a large S wave in lead I and a Q wave in lead III with T wave inversion in the same lead. Sometimes in addition there is T wave inversion in the chest leads over the right ventricle (V_1 to V_3). If the diagnosis is not satisfactorily established on clinical grounds it is a relatively simple procedure to perform right ventricular angiography. The latter will prove or disprove the diagnosis and at the same time give good anatomical definition of the embolic site or sites. For this reason this investigation is the one of choice when the diagnosis must be proved.

The important decision is whether the immediate degree of obstruction to blood flow is so great that there is not time to allow intensive medical thrombolytic therapy to take effect. If this is so, the operation of pulmonary embolectomy is indicated. If the circulation appears reasonable in the short term then the patient is treated with either heparinisation or thrombolytic therapy. At the present time it appears that thrombolytic therapy by streptokinase or urokinase may successfully lyse the clot if the patient survives long enough and does not sustain further emboli.

Details of thrombolytic therapy

1 Prednisolone 25 mg is given by intramuscular injection twice daily to guard against the risk of a sensitivity or anaphylactic reaction to streptokinase.

2 Intravenous administration of 600 000 i.u. of streptokinase in 100 ml of 5 % dextrose over a period of 30 minutes gives an initial loading dose which neutralises any anti-streptokinase antibodies which may be present due to previous streptococcal infections.

3 A maintenance dose of streptokinase is given at the rate of 100 000 i.u. per hour by infusing 540 ml of 5 % dextrose or normal saline, to which 600 000 i.u. of streptokinase have been added, every 6 hours over a period of 72 hours.

4 Anticoagulation is initiated at the end of this period by either giving oral anticoagulants such as phenindione (Dindevan) or warfarin during the last 24 hours of thrombolytic therapy or better, by giving intravenous heparin 4 hours after the end of the thrombolytic therapy. Anticoagulation should be continued until the patient is fully mobile and all the acute symptoms and signs have completely resolved.

Once the diluted solution of streptokinase is made up it should be used within 12 hours. Contraindications to thrombolytic therapy are any pre-existing risk of haemorrhage including defective haemostatic mechanisms, active peptic ulceration, severe systemic hypertension and cerebrovascular haemorrhage. Ideally it should not be used within 3 days following any operative procedure.

At the same time as the diagnosis is being established investigations to localise the site of the venous thrombosis from which the embolus has originated should be performed. These will enable accurate local surgical procedures to be carried out, if necessary, to prevent any further emboli.

General considerations in cardiovascular malfunction

When cardiovascular failure occurs, several of the previously considered factors are always involved. There may be a single precipitating cause (e.g. septicaemia producing toxic damage to the myocardium) but subsequently and often very rapidly other deleterious factors play an important additional part (e.g. dysrhythmias, hypovolaemia and acidosis).

When a low output ensues, a vicious circle of 'irreversibility' can develop owing to increasing involvement of other detrimental factors. The great majority of cases of 'irreversible shock' are due to delayed recognition and inadequate treatment of all the factors causing the failure. Intensive care of the failing cardiovascular system aims at maintaining an adequate cardiac output of blood of satisfactory quality. At the same time, treatment of the precipitating cause of the failure enables the system to regain intrinsic control such that supportive therapy is no longer necessary.

Although there are many causes of cardiovascular failure, the management of the failure itself has a common function with very little variation in individual cases. The common denominator in the majority of these cases is inadequate cardiac output and the primary aim is to improve the output.

Management of low cardiac output

When a patient is in an ICU a low cardiac output should always be recognised at an early stage and subsequently its trends closely monitored. The important signs of a reducing cardiac output are:

1 decreasing urine flow due to decreasing renal blood flow (see page 112);
2 increasing core-toe temperature gradient due to decreasing peripheral perfusion (see page 52);
3 increasing arterio-venous oxygen difference due to increased oxygen extraction by the tissues from the slowly flowing blood;

4 increasing tendency to acidosis due to poor tissue oxygenation (see page 00);
5 mental deterioration, the patient becoming confused, disorientated, semi-conscious and finally unconcious due to inadequate cerebral perfusion and oxygenation.

The blood pressure and the CVP may be low, normal or high and not directly relevant to recognition of low cardiac output. Recognition of the primary cause of the failure is important as this may allow specific treatment of the precipitating factor. The main aim of intensive care of the cardiovascular system is to improve the low cardiac output.

The general approach can be outlined in sequential steps, the specific details of which are discussed in the relevant parts of this book:

(a) Continually check and correct any acidosis and ensure that the arterial blood is satisfactory in respect to haemoglobin concentration and oxygen and carbon dioxide contents.

(b) Correct or control any dysrhythmias.

(c) If the CVP is low or normal apply the '5 to 15 rule' (see page 10).

(d) If the CVP is above 15 cmH$_2$O (1.5 kPa) stimulate increased force of cardiac contraction by the use of inotropic drugs, e.g. isoprenaline, adrenaline and digoxin. Induce a diuresis to protect renal function and excrete any water overload.

(e) If despite the appropriate treatment the clinical features indicate that the cardiac output remains unsatisfactory, initiate peripheral vascular dilation by the use of drugs such as phentolamine (Rogitine), phenoxybenzamine and nitroprusside, ensuring at the same time that the CVP is maintained by intravenous transfusion. The intravenous inotropic drug infusion should be continued.

(f) In severe cardiovascular failure which is refractory to the intensive therapy, it is valuable to paralyse the patient, intubate the trachea and institute intermittent positive pressure ventilation (IPPV). This will reduce the total body oxygen demand, ensure adequate ventilation during the critical period and also enable higher concentrations of oxygen to be given.

(g) Finally if the cardiovascular failure is so severe that the patient remains in a state of critically low cardiac output, circulatory assistance by aortic counterpulsation should be considered. Aortic counterpulsation applied in this critical situation has been shown to be of definite benefit. Its only contraindication is the presence of significant aortic valve regurgitation. This complex method of treatment requires the retrograde insertion of a catheter (with a balloon at its end) via the femoral artery into the descending thoracic aorta (Fig. 2.19). This balloon-catheter is then attached to the counterpulsation machine. By very sensitive and accurate controls this machine rapidly and actively both distends (with helium or carbon dioxide gas) and collapses the balloon in the aorta, such that the resistance to ejection of blood from the left ventricle into the aorta is reduced and coronary blood flow during cardiac diastole is increased.

Both these beneficial effects can tip the balance to allow reversal of the vicious circle of low cardiac output (see page 202).

Monitoring techniques

The purpose of patient monitoring is to afford early recognition of any instability or failure of the cardiovascular system and also to allow assessment of the response to treatment.

As intensive care techniques improve, monitoring becomes more sophisticated. In some ICUs the incorporation of a micro-processor into the system allows virtually continual, second by second or heart-beat by heart-beat assessment of the patient. There is instantaneous recognition of any unsatisfactory state and immediate communication of this fact to

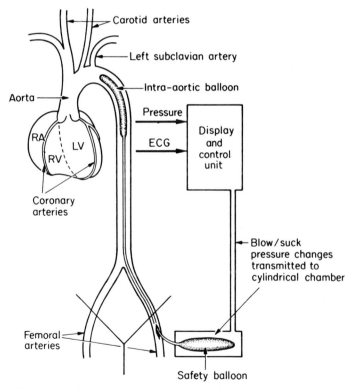

Fig. 2.19 (a) An intra-aortic balloon pump. The display unit shows a continuous ECG and the dynamic waveform of the radial artery and/or the pulmonary artery pressure. The balloon is set so that it pumps with every R wave or as few as 1:3 R waves

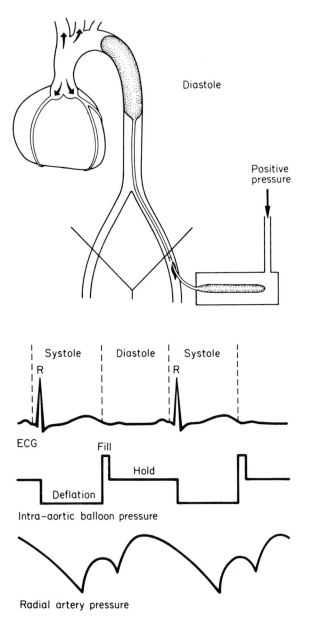

Fig. 2.19 (b) Ballon deflation is initiated by the R wave of each cardiac cycle and remains deflated for whatever time has been set by the operator on the control unit. The balloon then inflates and holds its inflation until the next R wave is received

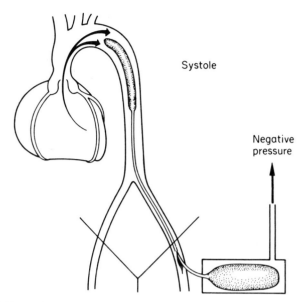

Fig. 2.19 (c) During diastole the balloon inflates to occlude the thoracic aorta so that blood is displaced retrogradely towards the brain and coronary arteries. With the following systole and subsequent deflation of the balloon a sucking effect occurs pulling the blood from the left ventricle into the aorta so decreasing the effort required of the left ventricle

the medical attendants. At the same time the computer facilities permit information correlation and trend assessment with instant information display at any time for any time period required.

Monitoring equipment also releases the nurse from the 'chore' of repeated measurements; the equipment can be expanded to enable it to chart its own readings. This gives the nurse more time to treat the patients, which is her major role. These instruments perform their monitoring function more rapidly and more frequently than could a doctor or nurse. It must be stressed that at no time does instrumentation replace the need for nursing and medical supervision, the instruments only make care easier and more efficient.

Routinely used measurements

1   Pressure measurements

(a) Central venous pressure (see page 9). Measurement of the CVP indicates measurement of the blood pressure in the right atrium or the venae cavae within the chest. To obtain the CVP it is necessary to insert a venous catheter into one of these structures. The most convenient entry point into the venous system is the median basilic vein in the antecubital fossa and the majority of such catheterisations will successfully pass into the right atrium. The cephalic vein and the external jugular veins are much less satisfactory; frequently the catheter will not pass into the superior vena cava because of the angulations these veins exhibit during their anatomical course. Alternatively, catheterisation of the internal jugular or subclavian veins are satisfactory procedures. The latter is very stable and comfortable because the catheter is splinted in its course between the clavicle and the first rib. Percutaneous catheterisation of the relatively large internal jugular or subclavian veins is an excellent procedure in patients where the peripheral veins have already been utilised, or in the severely shocked patient with collapsed veins.

The correct positioning of the CVP cannula is essential and this can be confirmed by the respiratory 'swing' (pressure change with respiration). Overtransfusion and other serious complications have arisen due to the incorrect assumption that the CVP was low in cases where the catheter had penetrated the vein wall and passed into other tissues, such as the mediastinum or the pleura.

Technical details for subclavian and internal jugular percutaneous catheterisation

Subclavian vein

This vein is firmly held by connective tissue as it passes over the first rib behind the medial third of the clavicle. It joins the internal jugular vein to form the innominate vein behind the sternoclavicular joint. The subclavian artery lies above and behind the vein, being separated from it by the insertion of the scalenus anterior muscle into the first rib. The patient is placed in the supine position with the head turned to the opposite side. The foot of the bed may be elevated to produce distension of the vein and avoid any risk of air embolism. The skin is punctured just lateral to and below the mid-point of the clavicle. The needle is advanced at about a 15 degree angle to the long axis of the clavicle aiming at the sternoclavicular joint. The lower border of the clavicle should be located with the tip of the needle which is then advanced immediately below it until the vein is entered. The catheter can then be passed through the needle into the subclavian vein and from there via the innominate vein into the superior vena cava and the right atrium (Fig. 2.20).

Internal jugular vein

This vein lying deep to the sterno-mastoid muscle has a very constant anatomical position and in the head down position has a diameter of approximately 2.5 cm. The position of the patient is the same as for subclavian vein catheterisation. The skin is punctured 3 cm above the

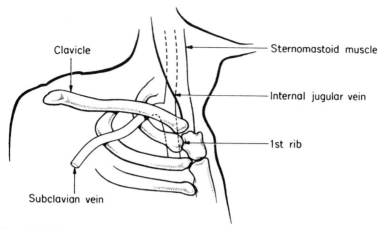

Fig. 2.20 Diagrams indicating the technique of percutaneous catheterisation of the internal jugular and subclavian veins

clavicle on the lateral border of the sternomastoid. The needle is aimed at the suprasternal notch and advanced under the sternomastoid until the vein is entered. The right side is preferred because of the danger of injury to the thoracic duct on the left. The carotid artery lies medially and deep to the vein. Other techniques for entering the internal jugular vein are also used.

There are many risks associated with internal jugular catheterisation and relate mainly to damage to the artery, thoracic duct or the phrenic nerve. There is a higher complication rate in subclavian vein catheterisation including pneumothorax, haemothorax, arterial damage and brachial plexus injury, but these can be avoided by a careful technique. The size and high flow rates in these two veins make them tolerant of a catheter for long periods of time.

In the sick infant central venous monitoring is even more essential but catheterisation is more difficult. It is usually best to perform a cut-down in these patients, and to ensure that an adequate size catheter can be inserted, the external jugular or long saphenous veins should be utilised. If these veins are exposed near their termination direct manipulation will enable the catheter to pass into the subclavian or common femoral veins respectively and then with ease to the right atrium.

Catheters
Polytetrafluoroethylene (PTFE, Teflon) catheters have good biological resistant properties and cause little tissue reaction. Radio-opaque catheters which can be visualised on X-ray are also preferred.

Some systems have the needle around the catheter, which is protected by a plastic splint. Despite these precautions, instances of catheters shearing to form emboli into the heart and lungs have been reported. A needle that can be withdrawn through the lumen of the catheter is much safer.

Central catheterisation via the median basilic vein at the ante-cubital fossa requires a 30 or 60 cm catheter. The route via the subclavian or internal jugular veins requires only a 20 cm catheter.

It is important to use an adequate diameter catheter to allow satisfactory pressure transmission. The catheter tip should lie within the chest in the vena cavae or right atrium. If the catheter tip is outside the chest the pressure measurements are artificially high and are not reliable. If inserted too far the catheter tip may come to rest in the right ventricle. This produces falsely high readings but the large pressure swings on the manometer usually make the diagnosis obvious. In practice the res-piratory swing of the intrathoracic venous pressure is a simple observa-tion which ensures that the catheter is both patent and within the chest. This observation should always be checked each time the venous pressure is read. To assume that a venous catheter impacted at the root of the neck is giving reliable and accurate pressure readings is completely unfounded and dangerous. The importance of venous pressure measurement in the intensive care patient is so great that there is no room for poor technique or guesswork.

Insertion of venous catheters is best performed with full sterile surgical precautions including skin cleaning, cap, mask and gloves and a sterile trolley to work from. Inserting a catheter in a surgically dirty manner is risking early phlebitis, venous thrombosis and bacteraemia. The skin entry site of the catheter should always be kept clean, dry and protected with a light dry dressing. Once the catheter has been positioned it should not be inserted further at a later date during 'manipulations'. This will always carry bacteria into the vein and greatly increase the risk of infection. If manipulation of the catheter becomes necessary, because the tip has become impacted against the caval or atrial wall, this should always be performed by cleaning the insertion site and then withdrawing the catheter by a short distance. It appears that the spread of bacteria along a venous catheter is from the cutaneous puncture site along the outside of the catheter rather than along its lumen (which is being continually flushed). This bacterial spread is virtually inevitable after 3 or 4 weeks and because of this a central venous catheter should always be replaced by a new one from a new site before this time. Insertion of a catheter by a poor technique can be associated with bacterial contami-nation of the tip within 48 hours. The bacterial spread can be further discouraged by placing the skin puncture site as far as reasonably possible from the vein entry site. It is clear from these facts that a percutaneous venous puncture is to be preferred to a cut-down whenever possible.

Having obtained central venous catheterisation the simplest method of monitoring the pressure is by means of a vertical glass water manometer as is used for CSF spinal manometry. This should be attached to the central venous line by a side arm controlled by a three-way tap (Fig. 10.5). When recording venous pressure trends it does not matter where the

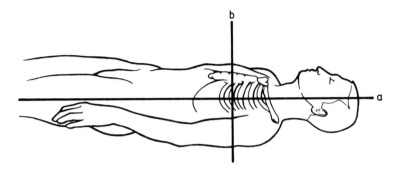

Fig. 2.21 The phlebostatic axis which is the point where a frontal plane (a), passing midway between the xiphoid and the dorsum of the body, transects a transverse plane (b) at the level of the 4th intercostal space

reference point for zero is taken on the patient's body as long as it is a constant with reference to the heart and the manometer. In this book the pressures referred to are the usual figures gained with a zero reference point at the phlebostatic axis, (Fig. 2.21) which passes through the posterior part of the atria and gives a constant venous pressure when the patient is moved from lying to sitting but is affected if the patient is turned. The sternal angle (Angle of Louis), or the midclavicular point are used as zero reference points in some units.

Measurement of the venous pressure by means of an electromagnetic transducer is more sophisticated and because of the increased sensitivity of the system allows measurement of the phasic pressures as well as the mean pressure. Also such a system can be coupled to a display or recording system. However, monitoring by means of a water manometer is satisfactory. Since pressure variations of as little as 5 cmH$_2$O can be significant, it is important that accurate levelling of the bottom of the water manometer, or the transducer, with the phlebostatic axis point of the patient (marked with a skin pencil) is maintained. A fluid levelling tube or a spirit level should be used for this purpose and not rough visual estimation. The levelling should be checked at frequent intervals to ensure that movement of the patient has not altered the alignment which would give false venous pressure readings.

(b) Left atrial pressure. In practice although the left atrial (LA) pressure may differ from the right atrial (RA) pressure in absolute values it is only rarely (in paediatric open-heart surgery for instance) that the two values do not fluctuate and trend in a similar manner. This applies even in left ventricular failure but is not valid in the presence of mitral valve disease. Indirect catheterisation of the left atrium is difficult and only after open-heart surgery is it sometimes monitored, the catheter being directly inserted into the left atrium during the operation. Recently the balloon-tipped flow-directed right heart catheter, Swan-Ganz, which can be

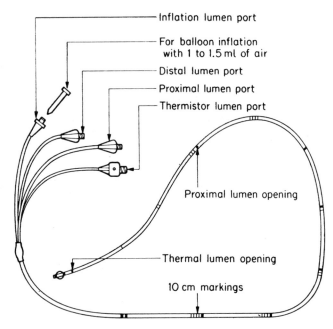

Inflation lumen port

For balloon inflation
with 1 to 1.5 ml of air

Distal lumen port

Proximal lumen port

Thermistor lumen port

Proximal lumen opening

Thermal lumen opening

10 cm markings

Fig. 2.22(a) Size 7 French gauge 110 cm four-lumen Swan-Ganz thermodilution catheter

introduced into the branches of the pulmonary artery via a peripheral vein, has proved useful (Fig. 2.22). When the catheter has passed as far as the right atrium, distension of the small balloon with 1.5 ml air or CO_2 results in the catheter being swept by the blood flow into the right ventricle and then onwards into a branch of one of the pulmonary arteries. With the balloon inflated in this position the pressure reading (the 'wedge' pressure) obtained is equivalent to the LA pressure. The catheter can be left *in situ* with the balloon deflated and LA pressure readings can be obtained as often as required by reinflating the balloon. If LA pressures are necessary this is the safest indirect method. Although these catheters are fairly expensive they should not be re-used.

(c) Arterial pressures. Arterial systolic and diastolic pressures can be measured indirectly in the usual manner by a sphygmomanometer. The sensitivity of this system is not great enough to enable accurate measurement of very low blood pressures with small pulse pressures, and when accurate recordings are most needed they are least reliable. The same criticism applies to all other methods of indirect blood pressure measurements. If a patient's condition is so poor that the blood pressure cannot be recorded accurately by the usual method it is important to gain direct measurement. This is most conveniently obtained by introducing a

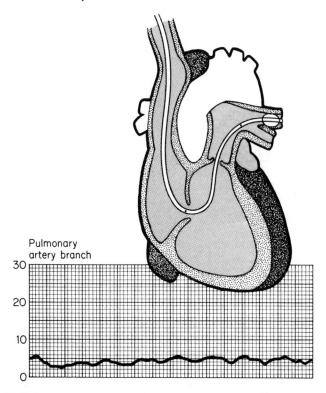

Fig. 2.22(b) Pulmonary artery balloon catheter wedged in a branch of the pulmonary artery showing typical wedge pressure recording (5 mmHg in this tracing)

cannula into the radial artery at the wrist. This can usually be done by percutaneous puncture, making a cut-down unnecessary. It is only necessary to introduce the catheter for a distance of approximately one inch. Further insertion of the catheter would unnecessarily obstruct radial artery branches. In the child it is best to perform a cut-down, and in the infant careful dissection also enables a satisfactorily sized catheter to be inserted at the same site.

The arterial pressure can be measured by attaching the cannula to a simple type of aneroid gauge (e.g. Tycos or Pressureveil). This will register only the mean arterial pressure but increasing or decreasing pressure trends are easily observed on the gauge dial. Preferably, by attaching the intra-arterial cannula to a pressure transducer the phasic pressures can be monitored and displayed on an oscilloscope screen or on a permanent record. The electromanometric measurement of arterial pressures, although involving expensive equipment, is very valuable. The system can display systolic, diastolic, pulse or mean pressures as required. The system is so sensitive that very low blood pressures are accurately measured. The accuracy of all pressure measuring systems, whether of the gauge or the electromanometer kind, must be verified before use.

An intra-arterial system of monitoring can be maintained for many days, but it is important that the catheter system be filled with heparinised saline at all times. The system should be gently flushed every hour with 1 ml of heparinised saline or used in conjunction with a pressurised, slow, continuous flushing system. This ensures that no blood enters the catheter system to cause thrombotic obstruction and loss of pressure wave transmission. Once the catheter has become blocked it is possible to clear it by pressure flushing, but patency is thereafter definitely limited.

A further advantage of arterial cannulation is the ease of access for arterial blood samples for blood-gas analysis and acid-base measurement. This is a better method of arterial blood sampling than repeated arterial punctures. The necessity of performing the latter often discourages the doctor from performing sufficient blood-gas estimations in conditions of cardiovascular stress. After samples are taken the catheter system is flushed clean of all blood with heparinised saline.

2   Urinary output

Most patients who are in acute low cardiac output should have bladder catheterisation with hourly measurements of urinary output. Apart from the importance of collecting all urine for volumetric and electrolytic balance estimations, urine excretion in the presence of normal renal function is dependent on adequate renal blood flow. Renal perfusion is maintained during early cardiovascular failure at the expense of perfusion of the extremities. As long as there is reasonable renal function, in the presence of normal kidneys, it can be assumed that in the short term there is adequate perfusion to the other vital centres (i.e. heart and brain). This does not mean the cardiac output is optimal.

The production of inadequate volumes of urine under these conditions indicates a critically low cardiac output causing pre-renal failure. If in the adult it is accepted that 700 ml is the lowest reasonable 24-hourly urine volume to maintain renal excretory compensation, then it can be said that a urine excretion of less than an average of 30 ml per hour is unacceptable. In practice, treatment is initiated if the urine volume is less than an average of 30 ml per hour over any 2 or 3 hour period. If the urine output falls below this rate further attention is directed towards increasing the cardiac output. At the same time a diuretic is given. The administration of frusemide or mannitol has a protective effect on kidney hypoxia by stimulating increased urine flow and increased afferent renal blood flow.

3   Core-toe temperature

In conditions of cardiovascular stress there is an early response by reduction of perfusion to the extremities. This is produced by peripheral vasoconstriction which directs a larger proportion of the falling cardiac output to the vital organs, such as heart, brain, kidneys and liver. In severe low output states the vasoconstriction produces palpably cold and visibly pale extremities. If central (e.g. rectal) and peripheral (e.g. toe) temperatures are monitored by thermistor probes, a very sensitive assessment of the peripheral circulation is obtained. A patient in full cardiac compensation lying in a comfortable ambient temperature will have a toe temperature approximately 1°C lower than the rectal temperature. Within a few minutes of the onset of even a mild cardiovascular stress (brisk bleeding of 100 to 200 ml of blood in the adult) the toe temperature shows a significant fall. The resulting core-toe temperature gradient is a sensitive indirect indication of the circulatory state. A decreasing cardiac output will result in an increasing core-toe temperature gradient and a subsequent increasing cardiac output will result in a decreasing temperature gradient (Fig. 2.23).

4   Electrocardiogram

Any variation in the heart from sinus rhythm results in decreasing cardiac efficiency. The immediate recognition of any dysrhythmia is important. The earlier a dysrhythmia is recognised the more likely the treatment will be successful and the less likely the cardiovascular effect will be detrimental. For this monitoring purpose it is necessary to have only two or three precordial chest electrodes, which are easily maintained and comfortable for the patient.

5   Blood gases

Measurement of these parameters requires the use of a blood-gas analyser (page 92). The heparinised blood sample should be immediately processed after it has been taken. Exposure of the blood sample to air is avoided. It can be stored in an airtight container in a mixture of ice and water (0°C) but under circumstances of intensive care storage of the sample indicates that the measurement was unnecessary in the first place.

It is usual to take an arterial rather than a venous specimen as the oxygen and carbon dioxide gas tensions will give an indication of lung function. If in addition a central venous specimen of blood is analysed (or better still a sample taken from a pulmonary artery catheter), the difference of the oxygen tension between the arterial and venous bloods indicates the degree of oxygen extraction from the blood by the tissues. If the cardiac output is low there will be a slow circulation and tissue oxygen extraction will be greater than if the circulation were normal. The arterio-venous oxygen difference is therefore another indirect indication of the circulatory state. In practice the core-toe temperature gradient has replaced this method because of its greater simplicity of reproduction for monitoring purposes. The arterial blood gas analysis remains, however,

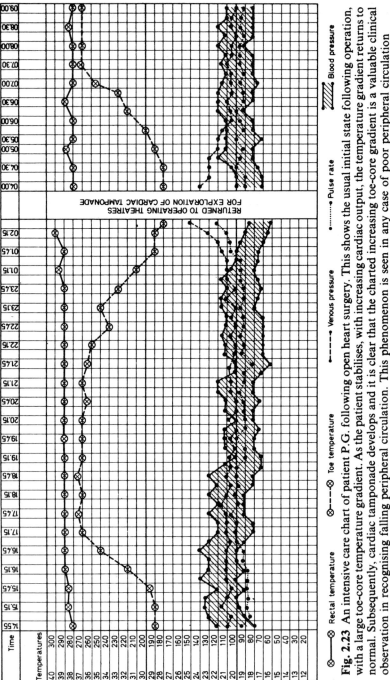

Fig. 2.23 An intensive care chart of patient P.G. following open heart surgery. This shows the usual initial state following operation, with a large toe-core temperature gradient. As the patient stabilises, with increasing cardiac output, the temperature gradient returns to normal. Subsequently, cardiac tamponade develops and it is clear that the charted increasing toe-core gradient is a valuable clinical observation in recognising falling peripheral circulation. This phenomenon is seen in any case of poor peripheral circulation.

an important investigation for assessment of the acid-base balance and of respiratory function.

6   Haemoglobin and haematocrit

These are basic and important investigations of the oxygen carrying power of the blood and in severe bleeding these measurements will be repeatedly necessary.

7   Chest X-ray, serum electrolytes, blood urea, urinary electrolytes, urea excretion and blood and urine osmolarities

These are also investigated regularly in patients undergoing intensive care to gain further information regarding the internal environment.

8   Other monitoring equipment

As electronic equipment has grown more sophisticated with greater reliability and stability, more monitoring facilities have become available. These include:

Dysrhythmia monitor
This equipment, used in conjunction with the electrocardiogram, can recognise and count any type of nodal or ventricular extra-systole. The machine can be programmed to set off an alarm if the extrasystolic rate rises above a predetermined number per minute, giving warning of increasing myocardial instability.

Memory loop
This is an electromagnetic tape loop continually recording the electro-cardiogram and storing this for a period of usually 10 seconds. Should a cardiac arrest occur, the electromagnetic recording of the electro-cardiogram immediately before the arrest can then be played back and the rhythm immediately before the arrest analysed.

Trend recorder
This machine records any selected physiological parameter such as pulse rate, blood pressure or extrasystoles. The machine records the readings at fixed intervals on a slowly moving length of graph paper or the information can be stored in an oscilloscope. The intervals are usually every minute. Any slow trend over a period of minutes to hours is easily appreciated, for example increasing pulse rate or dropping blood pressure. Appropriate treatment can then be initiated to stop any detrimental trend. This machine can release the nurse from the time-consuming necessity of recording the basic physiological parameters on the traditional intensive care chart (Appendix VI).

3

The Respiratory System

Physiological considerations

Although the term respiration is more correctly used to describe the exchange of gases between the cells and the environment, it is commonly applied to external respiration or breathing, which is the first stage of this process. Respiration or breathing is therefore the mechanical method by which air is taken into the lungs (inspiration) and then let out again (expiration). The prime purpose of breathing is to provide the body tissues with sufficient oxygen for their needs and at the same time to excrete carbon dioxide, one of the waste products of metabolism.

The rate and depth of respiration are adjusted to the requirements at any particular time and are controlled by a diffuse collection of cells (the 'respiratory centre') in the medulla and pons of the brain and by the peripheral chemical receptors (chemoreceptors) in the carotid bodies. The pattern of respiration is also influenced by afferent nervous impulses from receptors in the skin, larynx, carotid bodies, great vessels, heart and lungs. Anxiety may also produce an increase in rate.

Under normal conditions, the level of carbon dioxide in the blood is the most important factor, and a rise will stimulate breathing. The converse is also true. Normally oxygen levels have little effect, unless the respiratory centre has become insensitive to carbon dioxide as in chronic respiratory disease. If this occurs, low oxygen levels will then stimulate breathing via the peripheral chemoreceptors in the carotid bodies.

Ventilation

The volume of breathing or *pulmonary ventilation* depends also on the efficient function of the respiratory muscles (intercostal muscles and diaphragm) and the integrity of the rib cage.

Inspiration occupies approximately one-third of the respiratory cycle while expiration takes up the remaining two-thirds. During this sequence, a volume of gas is moved in and out of the lungs. The inspired gas is normally air and the volume is known as the *tidal volume*. This volume varies according to the size of the patient but is usually 350–500 ml at rest or about 7 ml/kg body weight. Expired air contains 3–4 % carbon dioxide compared with 0.03 % in inspired air. The oxygen content is only 16–17 % compared with 21 % in inspired air. Instead of percentages we often express gas concentrations as fractions; an FIO_2 of 0.21 means a fractional inspired oxygen concentration of 0.21 (i.e. 21 %). Only about two-thirds of the tidal volume is involved in the gas exchange process taking place in the alveoli. This is termed the effective or *alveolar ventilation*. The remainder is referred to as the *physiological dead space* which is composed of two components—the *anatomical dead space* and the *alveolar dead space*. The anatomical dead space is the volume of the conducting airways such as the mouth, trachea and bronchi, and is approximately 3 ml/kg body weight. The alveolar dead space is a further volume of gas in the alveoli where gas exchange does not take place.

The volume of air remaining in the lungs at the end of a normal expiration is called *functional residual capacity* (FRC). In normal subjects, FRC is affected by posture which influences the resting position of the chest wall; because of this the FRC is about 25 % less when the patient is in a supine position than in an upright position. Since the FRC is the lung volume into which the inspired gas is mixed, it acts as a buffer or a reserve of oxygen to some extent. This reserve is depleted in any situation in which FRC is reduced.

The *minute volume* is obtained by multiplying the tidal volume by the respiratory rate, and is usually in the range of 4–6 litres. The *vital capacity* (VC) is easily measured and can give an assessment of airway obstruction when measured over a timed period. It is the total of the inspiratory reserve volume, tidal volume and expiratory reserve volume. The residual air can never be expelled (Fig. 3.1).

Compliance

In order to draw air into the lungs, the respiratory muscles must overcome the elastic recoil of the lungs and the resistance of the airways. Compliance is a term relating pressure and volume changes and is a measure of the

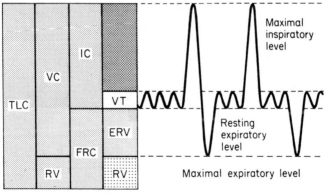

TLC	total lung capacity	FRC	functional residual capacity
VC	vital capacity	VT	tidal volume
RV	residual volume	ERV	expiratory reserve volume
IC	inspiratory capacity		

Fig. 3.1 Lung volumes

'stiffness' of the lungs. It is expressed by the ratio:

$$\frac{\text{volume change produced}}{\text{pressure change required}}$$

A low compliance therefore implies a situation in which a high pressure is required to produce a given volume change. The opposite will also be true; if only a small pressure is required to produce the same increase in volume, then the lungs are said to have a high compliance. Total thoracic (C_T) compliance is the combined measurement of chest wall (C_{CW}) and lung (C_L) components and is approximately 100 ml/cmH$_2$O. The relationship is:

$$\frac{1}{C_{CW}} + \frac{1}{C_L} = \frac{1}{C_T}$$

Since in health the values of C_L and C_{CW} are about the same, namely 200 ml/cm H$_2$O,

$$\frac{1}{200} + \frac{1}{200} = 0.01 \ \text{l/cmH}_2\text{O} \ (\text{i.e. } 100 \ \text{ml/cmH}_2\text{O})$$

To compare individuals of different sizes, the values of C_T, C_L and C_{CW} must be standardised. This is done by dividing the compliance by some specific lung volume such as the FRC to give the *specific compliance* (sC). The value of sC is about 0.08/cm H$_2$O.

Oxygen

For efficient function, the respiratory mechanism must be capable of maintaining the tension of oxygen (Po_2) in the arterial blood at its normal value of approximately 100 mmHg (13.3 kPa) when breathing air. At the same time, the carbon dioxide tension (Pco_2) should be maintained at a level of approximately 40 mmHg (5.3 kPa). Any marked deviation from these figures will produce a disturbance of the normal chemical process with a resulting change of acidity of the blood. This is normally very accurately controlled at pH 7.4 (7.36–7.44). In chronic respiratory disease, where the arterial Pco_2 is above normal, compensatory mechanisms are brought into action in an attempt to preserve a normal blood pH.

When oxygen comes into contact with blood by diffusing through the alveolar membrane, it will reversibly combine with the haemoglobin of the red blood cells to form oxyhaemoglobin. In addition a very small amount, 0.3 ml/100 ml, will dissolve in the plasma. As each gram of haemoglobin can carry 1.39 ml of oxygen (sometimes 1.34 ml is quoted instead), 100 ml of blood with a haemoglobin level of 14 g/100 ml is capable of carrying approximately 20 ml of oxygen. The haemoglobin is normally 100% saturated only when the arterial Po_2 is between 250 and 700 mmHg (33–93 kPa). Breathing room air (21% oxygen) produces an arterial Po_2

of about 90–100 mmHg (12–13 kPa) with a haemoglobin saturation of 95–98 %. At a P_{O_2} of 60 mmHg (8.0 kPa) the blood is 90 % saturated, but below this the saturation falls steeply for any drop in oxygen tension.

The normal O_2 dissociation or association curve. The shape of the oxyhaemoglobin dissociation (or association) curve for normal adult blood at 37°C and at pH 7.40 is shown in Fig. 3.2. At P_{O_2} of 100 mmHg (the 'arterial point') haemoglobin is 97.5 % saturated. Therefore, increasing the P_{O_2} will not add much more oxygen to the haemoglobin and most of the additional oxygen goes only into solution. Full saturation occurs at about 250 mmHg (33 kPa) P_{O_2}.

There is very little change in saturation (and therefore the amount of oxygen associated with haemoglobin) between P_{O_2} levels of 70 mmHg and 100 mmHg. The lower portion of the S-shaped curve (Fig. 3.2) is concerned with the release of oxygen. The curve is very steep between 10 mmHg and 40 mmHg, and the mixed venous point $P\bar{v}_{O_2}$ is shown as 40 mmHg. At this point haemoglobin is still 75 % saturated but at a P_{O_2} of 10 mmHg only 9.6 % is left as an oxygen reserve. The steep slope of the curve implies that the tissues are protected because they are able to withdraw large amounts of oxygen from the blood for relatively small decreases in P_{O_2}.

The 'affinity' of haemoglobin is characterised by the point marked P_{50} which allows easy comparisons between various dissociation curves. P_{50} is the oxygen partial pressure at which 50 % of the haemoglobin is saturated. Normally (at 37°C, pH 7.40, P_{CO_2} 40 mmHg or 5.3 kPa and a normal haemoglobin concentration) the P_{50} is 27 mmHg or 3.6 kPa. If the

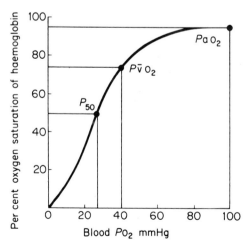

Fig. 3.2 The relationship between blood oxygen tension (P_{O_2}) and oxygen saturation of haemoglobin

affinity of the haemoglobin for oxygen changes, then the oxyhaemoglobin dissociation curve will change its position—a process known as 'shifting' the curve.

The shape of the oxyhaemoglobin dissociation curve can change quite markedly if either the microenvironment or the chemistry of the red blood cells is altered, or if the blood contains abnormal forms of haemoglobin. Thus both the uptake and the unloading of oxygen from haemoglobin can be affected. A decrease in oxygen affinity results in a shift to the right; thus at any given P_{O_2} there is a decrease in saturation, aiding oxygen movement from blood to tissues. However, although oxygen unloading from haemoglobin is enhanced there is less oxygen loaded onto the haemoglobin as the blood passes through the lungs. Shifts of the dissociation curve to the right are due to a raised P_{CO_2}, lowered pH, hyperpyrexia and an increase in concentration of the 2,3-diphosphogly-cerate (2,3-DPG) enzyme in the red blood cells. A shift of the dissociation curve to the left means that haemoglobin is less able to release oxygen and this is due to hypothermia, alkalosis (low P_{CO_2} or raised pH) or a reduction in 2,3-DPG. A common cause of low 2,3-DPG is transfusion of old blood, particularly that which has been stored with citrate as an anticoagulant (Fig. 3.3).

The result of insufficient oxygenation of the tissues is *hypoxia*. The term *anoxia* is sometimes used, but strictly speaking this implies complete and absolute absence of oxygen in the tissues and is therefore inaccurate. *Hypoxaemia* is a more specific term implying a low oxygen saturation of

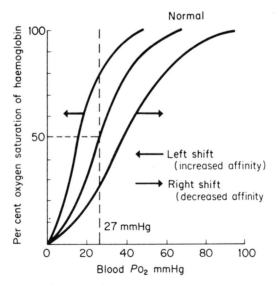

Fig. 3.3 Shifts in the oxyhaemoglobin dissociation curve resulting from changes in the oxygen affinity of haemoglobin

blood. In addition to respiratory causes, anaemia, circulatory stagnation and toxic disturbances of the enzyme systems will all produce hypoxaemia. Fortunately, most organs will function as long as the oxygen saturation is 50 % (P_{O_2} 30 mmHg), but below this figure sustained life is unlikely.

The bluish colour of the skin associated with hypoxaemia is termed *cyanosis*. It is closely related to the amount of reduced or non-oxygenated haemoglobin in the blood. Generally at least 5 g of reduced haemoglobin must be present for this to be clinically apparent. If, however, the patient is polycythaemic with a high haemoglobin level, 5 g of reduced haemoglobin may be present even with a satisfactory oxygen saturation. Conversely, an anaemic patient with a haemoglobin level of only 6 g will not show cyanosis even if 50 % of the haemoglobin is in the reduced form as this will amount to only 3 g. Nevertheless, cyanosis is normally a good practical guide to oxygenation. With uniform colour-corrected lighting, the experienced eye can usually make a decision as to whether the patient is hypoxic or not. The lips are a better guide than the ears as stagnation may produce a false impression. For this reason, poor circulatory states may give the appearance of cyanosis in the presence of adequate blood oxygenation. This is termed *peripheral* cyanosis as distinct from the true or *central* cyanosis. Nevertheless, it is a good maxim to consider cyanosis to be a sign of hypoxaemia until proved otherwise, for instance by measurement of P_{O_2}.

Oxygen flux (available oxygen). The available oxygen is the quantity of oxygen available for utilisation by the body and is calculated from the cardiac output and from the amount of oxygen carried by each ml of blood:

$$\begin{array}{lll} \text{available} = & \text{cardiac} \times & \text{arterial} \\ \text{oxygen} & \text{output} & \text{oxygen content} \\[4pt] \text{(ml O}_2\text{/min)} & \text{(ml blood/min)} & \text{(ml O}_2\text{/ml blood)} \end{array}$$

Typical figures for a cardiac output of 5000 ml/min and an arterial oxygen content of 0.2 ml O_2/ml blood (i.e. 20 ml O_2/100 ml blood) give an available oxygen of 1000 ml/min. A conscious resting patient uses at least 250 ml/min of this available oxygen. The circulating blood therefore loses 25 % of its oxygen (250/1000 ml) so leaving the mixed venous blood returning to the lungs via the pulmonary artery 75 % saturated. This 75 % of unextracted oxygen forms an oxygen reserve which can be called upon in stress conditions.

Carbon dioxide

So far the discussion has concerned oxygen, but the partial pressure or tension of carbon dioxide (P_{CO_2}) in the blood similarly bears a relationship to the concentration of carbon dioxide in the inspired gas mixture. Under normal conditions, compensatory ventilatory changes occur which maintain the P_{CO_2} at a normal level. These are initiated by the action of special chemoreceptors which in turn stimulate or depress respiration.

In the case of carbon dioxide, diffusion is in the reverse direction to oxygen. As carbon dioxide is very soluble, it diffuses rapidly across the alveolar membrane. For this reason, it is only disturbances of ventilation that are usually responsible for marked alterations of P_{CO_2}.

Disturbances of ventilation

Hyperventilation (overbreathing) lowers the P_{CO_2} in the arterial blood. This condition of *hypocapnia* is not associated with a rise in P_{O_2} as the blood is fully saturated at the partial pressure of the inspired oxygen and overventilation cannot increase this. There is however, considerable increase in oxygen and energy requirement for the increased amount of work involved.

Hypoventilation (underbreathing) produces a rise in P_{CO_2} in the arterial blood. This condition of hypercapnia is usually associated with a fall in P_{O_2} as there is reduced alveolar ventilation.

Acidity and pH values

Acidity is measured as pH, which is a convenient way of expressing hydrogen ion concentration. pH is the negative logarithm of the hydrogen ion concentration, and therefore acid solutions with high hydrogen ion concentrations have a low pH; and alkaline solutions a high pH. Neutral solutions have a pH of 7.

$$\text{pH} \propto \frac{[HCO_3^-]}{P_{CO_2} \times \alpha}$$

where $[HCO_3^-]$ is the concentration of bicarbonate ions in plasma and α is the coefficient of solubility of CO_2 in plasma. If normal values are inserted we obtain:

$$\frac{[24]\ mmol/l}{40\ mmHg \times 0.03\ ml\ CO_2/mmHg}$$

or a ratio of 20:1

Hence, an increase in P_{CO_2} will increase the value of the denominator in the expression and hence the value of pH will fall. Bicarbonate will then be retained by the kidneys in an attempt to keep the pH normal. This situation is called *respiratory acidosis*. In hyperventilation, the P_{CO_2} will fall elevating the pH and producing an alkaline state of *respiratory alkalosis*.

Perfusion

Perfusion is a factor of vital importance in the production of a satisfactory blood gas state. This term refers to the supply and distribution of blood to the alveoli. The output of the heart and the patency of the vessels supplying the alveoli are factors influencing perfusion. Ventilation and perfusion must be adequately matched.

In Fig. 3.4, (a) shows the 'ideal' state where there is perfect ventilation matched by perfect perfusion and (b) shows an extreme situation where ventilation is very much reduced, either as a result of respiratory depression or obstruction in the airways. If perfusion of these alveoli is maintained, then oxygen cannot be taken up by the blood as it passes through the lung capillaries; hence, deoxygenated blood is transmitted to the left side of the circulation (pulmonary veins) and constitutes a 'right-to-left' *shunt* or *pulmonary venous admixture*. This 'blue' blood mixes with ('admixture') well-oxygenated blood returning from normally ventilated areas of the lung and thus the final degree of oxygenation of the mixture will lie somewhere between these two extremes. The exact amount of desaturation of the arterial blood on the left side of the circulation depends upon both the content of oxygen in the blood and the amount of blood returning from each source. If the degree of oxygenation of blood entering the lung from the pulmonary artery is already seriously impaired,

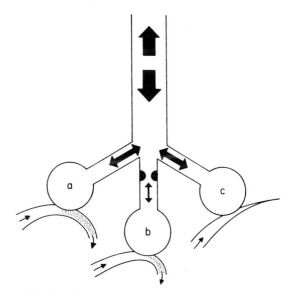

Fig. 3.4 Three states of ventilation and perfusion

then the effect of even a small amount of shunt will produce gross arterial desaturation.

Also in Fig. 3.4, (c) shows the third possibility where ventilation is normal but perfusion to that alveolus has virtually ceased. In such a situation there can be no gas exchange across the alveolar membrane no matter how good the ventilation. Because ventilation is wasted in this situation (i.e. it cannot do any good because there is no pulmonary blood flow in that area) the alveolus is called a *'dead space'* or *'dead air'* unit. The dead space can be calculated or measured by various techniques which include analysis of the arterial blood and of the composition of the gas entering and leaving the lungs. The *ratio* of the dead space to the tidal volume is used as an index of ventilatory inefficiency. This is of value in following the progress of a patient with respiratory failure. In healthy patients the ratio is about 0.3 for a 70 kg adult (i.e. 140/490 ml).

The ratio between alveolar ventilation (V) and perfusion (Q) is called the V/Q *ratio*. Although the examples cited above are extremes, there is a whole range of possibilities between normal and absent ventilation on the one hand, and perfusion on the other. Moreover, there is the possibility of abnormalities in both ventilation and perfusion simultaneously. To a certain extent this may be an advantage, because if the perfusion of the lung in the situation shown in Fig. 3.4 (b) is reduced then the amount of admixture will also be reduced and hence the extent of desaturation on the arterial side of the systemic circulation will be lessened. This is obviously a beneficial or protective mechanism. However, it has been shown that this mechanism is abolished in certain situations, as in some disease states and by certain anaesthetic drugs. The V/Q ratio of the lung as a whole is 0.8 in health (i.e. $V = 4$ l/min, $Q = 5$ l/min). However, the exact distribution of both ventilation and perfusion in the lung varies widely according to the position of the patient. In an upright person the 'top' of the lung has a V/Q ratio much greater than this (i.e. a low pulmonary flow towards the apices of the lung) whereas the 'bottom' of the lung has a lower V/Q ratio.

Disturbances of normal respiratory physiology

Depending upon their severity, disorders of the normal physiology produce varying degrees of failure of the respiratory system. Respiratory failure is one of the commonest conditions treated in the ICU. It has been defined on blood gas analysis as a P_{CO_2} greater than 50 mmHg (6.7 kPa) or a P_{O_2} less than 60 mmHg (8.0 kPa) when breathing air.

Causes of respiratory dysfunction may be grouped under the following headings although more than one group may contribute to the final result:

1 Ventilation defects
2 Perfusion defects
3 Diffusion defects

1 Ventilation defects

Reduction in tidal volume and therefore alveolar ventilation may be caused by a failure of the mechanics of breathing. This may be nervous, muscular, bony or pulmonary in origin. It is reflected by a lowering of the oxygen saturation and a rise in P_{CO_2} of the arterial blood.

The nervous system disturbances may be central or peripheral. The central nervous system may be damaged and its activity depressed by trauma, haemorrhage, thrombosis, hypoxia, hypotension or poisons. Overdosage of central nervous system depressant drugs is becoming a major cause of respiratory insufficiency. Barbiturates and other hypnotics form the major group of depressant drugs, although narcotics (morphine and pethidine) produce the same effect. The central nervous system may also be stimulated by drugs and toxins in such a way as to produce muscular rigidity and respiratory incoordination. Tetanus (page 156) is a classical example of this stimulation in which spasms of muscular contraction cause chest wall rigidity and severe hypoxia. Convulsions from epilepsy, encephalitis and strychnine poisoning produce similar effects.

Poliomyelitis (page 154) affects the anterior horn cells of the nerves to the intercostal muscles and diaphragm. This results in respiratory paralysis of varying degrees. Polyneuritis (page 154) may similarly produce respiratory paralysis by injury to the lower motor neurones. Botulism may give rise to respiratory paralysis due to a neurotoxin formed by the organism *Clostridium botulinus.*

Myasthenia gravis and muscle relaxant drugs (e.g. gallamine, d-tubocurarine and pancuronium) produce muscle paralysis by an action at the neuromuscular junction (page 155). By preventing transmission of the impulse from the nerves to the muscles of the thorax, varying degrees of respiratory insufficiency will result. Neuromuscular transmission may be blocked during treatment of myasthenia by excessive dosage of anticholinergic drugs. Pure muscle diseases seldom produce disturbances of pulmonary function. However, exhaustion in patients with severe respiratory or cardiac disease may produce underventilation due to lack of muscle power.

Damage to the bony thoracic cage may result in underventilation. If several ribs are fractured and there is an unstable segment, a 'flail chest' results (page 93). During inspiration the injured side is sucked in but the normal side expands in the usual way. On expiration the reverse takes place. This paradoxical respiration is seen only during spontaneous breathing and is abolished by intermittent positive pressure ventilation (IPPV). Poor ventilation and *paradoxical breathing* result in collapse and consolidation which further aggravate respiratory embarrassment. Pain from fractures, stab wounds and thoracotomy wounds may interfere with normal respiration. Over-energetic cardiac resuscitation producing rib fractures may contribute to this group.

Tension pneumothorax, bronchopleural fistula and diaphragmatic hernia in the newborn are all further cases where the mechanics of breathing are upset.

Pulmonary causes of underventilation usually occur as a result of airway obstruction at any point from the mouth to the terminal bronchioles. In the larger passages obstruction reduces the tidal volume, whereas in the smaller tubes constriction of the lumen will increase airway resistance and therefore reduce ventilation.

Obstruction may be due to tumours of the tongue, pharynx, larynx, trachea or bronchi. Reversible obstruction due to foreign bodies and secretions produces similar results. Inflammatory process of the larynx, trachea and bronchi may result in oedema and subsequent obstruction. Bronchospasm associated with asthma and chronic bronchitis will similarly narrow the small airways.

Reduction in alveolar ventilation will also occur in emphysema, interstitial pulmonary fibrosis, pneumoconiosis, pulmonary oedema and pneumonia.

2   Perfusion defects

The blood flow aspect of the ventilation/perfusion ratio is vital in the understanding of respiratory failure. This is shown diagrammatically on page 63 and in practice the most important situation is where the perfusion is normal but the ventilation is impaired. The result is similar to a right-to-left shunt with suboxygenation of the arterial blood. There are some instances where the perfusion is less than normal with normal ventilation. This is relatively unusual but may occur in embolism of the pulmonary artery or its branches by thrombus, gas (usually air) or fat. Pulmonary thromboembolism is the most common cause, and the situation is aggravated by reflex bronchoconstriction and low cardiac output. The blood gas picture is complicated by these, but the overall picture is one of hypoxia. Perfusion defects are also present in congenital heart disease with anomalies or disturbances of the pulmonary vasculature. They may also be a feature of the complex respiratory abnormalities following open-heart surgery, or as a result of the diseased processes in cor pulmonale and left ventricular failure.

In many pulmonary diseases, the causes of respiratory failure are several. As a result there is overlap from one group to another. For example, in pneumonia consolidation and collapse will cause shunting of blood through non-ventilated lung, while secretions will obstruct the airways and exudate interfere with diffusion.

3   Diffusion defects

These are less common than ventilation defects and although thickening of the alveolar wall might be thought to produce an obstruction to diffusion, the effects are probably due to impaired local ventilation. Nevertheless, pulmonary oedema or exudate from inhalation of irritant fumes (e.g. smoke and ammonia) must present some barrier to gas diffusion across the alveolar membrane. Other causes of such a diffusion block are carcinomatosis (with tumour infiltration of lymphatics in the lung) and beryllium poisoning. Some diffusion block may also be found in patients who survive the pulmonary acid-aspiration syndrome.

Intensive care of respiratory disturbances

Respiratory failure from any cause results in hypoxia and possibly carbon dioxide retention. The effects of the latter are not as serious as hypoxia, although the respiratory acidosis produced will further aggravate hypoxia. If this persists, a chain of events will ensue which, if not broken, will result in death. Fortunately, most organs can function as long as the oxygen saturation does not fall below 50 % but below this level cerebral, renal and hepatic failure result. Hypoxia must be treated urgently, and patients on the brink of respiratory failure treated energetically and observed meticulously.

The consequence of hypoxia is metabolic acidosis. Anaerobic metabolism of pyruvic acid to produce energy allows the accumulation of lactic acid. This acidotic state leads to reduced cardiac contraction and reduced blood flow. This in turn leads to further hypoxia. The respiratory acidosis from carbon dioxide retention will be a further strain on any compensating mechanisms. It can be seen that not only will oxygen be required but, if the hypoxia has existed for any length of time, sodium bicarbonate or other chemical buffers will be required to neutralise the acids. If untreated this cycle of events will end fatally.

Ventilation defects

These form the main groups of disorders leading to failure of the respiratory system. If they were pure ventilation defects, all that would be required would be to increase the tidal volume by artifically ventilating the lungs with air. In fact, as there are usually other factors present, such as infection with consolidation and collapse, added oxygen has to be given in addition to the artificial lung ventilation IPPV (see page 70). In myasthenic crisis or poliomyelitis, ventilation with air alone may be all that is required but usually the addition of some oxygen is necessary.

If added oxygen is given by a mask, the concentration of the oxygen is increased in the alveoli but this does not relieve the carbon dioxide retention. In fact, by increasing the oxygen at this stage one of the stimuli to breathing, namely hypoxia, has been removed. This may produce underventilation with further carbon dioxide retention. The respiratory centre may have become insensitive to high carbon dioxide levels. However, in some mild cases of respiratory failure, oxygen in carefully metered doses may be sufficient to avert the effects of hypoxia without carbon dioxide accumulating to an unacceptable level, remembering that some patients will be used to high P_{CO_2} levels.

As previously stated, there are usually many causes operating together, and ventilation with air will lower the P_{CO_2} without helping the low P_{O_2}. This may be due to 'shunting' of blood through non-ventilated atelectatic (collapsed) areas of lung. This is a clinical situation where the ventilation/perfusion ratio is disturbed. Shunting will occur until the collapsed alveoli are re-expanded or the pneumonic areas resolved. During spontaneous ventilation, there is evidence that the other alveoli may over-ventilate in a compensatory manner and help to prevent carbon dioxide retention. This mechanism would be insufficient in cases of severe respiratory failure. With IPPV the carbon dioxide level can easily be reduced and oxygen added to the inspired gases will raise the P_{O_2}. Although 100% oxygen should not be withheld in emergency hypoxic states, it should be remembered that high concentrations of oxygen given for any length of time will cause damage to the alveoli, and therefore cause further decompensation. Where possible, the concentration of oxygen should be carefully monitored with an oxygen analyser and, in addition, arterial P_{O_2} levels followed. Generally, about 30–40% oxygen is sufficient, but in severe lung damage much higher concentrations will be required. The inspired oxygen concentration should be reduced if the P_{O_2} exceeds 150 mm Hg (20 kPa).

In terms of ventilation/perfusion disorders, the conditions where there is reduced ventilation and relatively normal blood perfusion are postoperative atelectasis (from blood or mucus), bronchopneumonia, 'perfusion lung', oedematous and congested lungs (left ventricular failure), bronchial obstruction (tumours, foreign bodies), flail chest, thoracic limitation by pain, myasthenia, poliomyelitis, tetanus, drug overdose, brain damage, chest wounds, pneumothorax, asthma and other chronic respiratory disorders.

Ventilation in excess of perfusion

Oxygen tension cannot be raised without adding oxygen to the inspired mixture, as the blood will be saturated for that pressure of oxygen. The carbon dioxide may be normal or possibly raised. This situation does not occur in isolation clinically. It is, however, present in addition to ventilation defects, for example in pulmonary embolus and emphysema. Added oxygen in metered concentration is of help, but if the condition is severe IPPV will be required.

It is important to remember that the cause of respiratory failure may be multifactorial. Blood gases are the best guide to the line of treatment required. For example if the P_{CO_2} is normal and the P_{O_2} low, added oxygen in carefully measured amounts is all that is required provided that the patient is not fatigued. The increased work called upon by respiratory distress increases the oxygen requirement and puts an extra load on the respiratory and circulatory systems. This work is required to overcome resistance in narrow airways, lung stiffness and mucus obstruction. This extra load, which may be responsible for 40–50 % of oxygen consumption, will set up a cycle of events which may be broken only by IPPV (Fig. 3.5).

Fatigue may be the factor which determines whether artificial ventilation should be instigated. Respiratory distress, or 'breathlessness' is referred to as *dyspnoea*. It will accompany respiratory failure but may be the first sign of respiratory insufficiency when the compensatory mechanisms are battling to retain respiratory homeostasis. In this case it will prelude failure, and it is at this stage action should be taken.

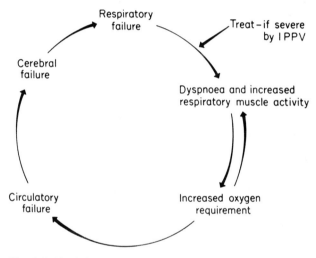

Fig. 3.5 The influence of respiratory failure on other systems

Diffusion defects

These are rare and, if they occur, the disorder is usually one of suboxygenation since carbon dioxide will readily diffuse even through a diseased alveolar membrane. Usually ventilation defects co-exist, and these will probably require correction by IPPV. Even when the alveolar membrane is damaged or covered with oedema fluid, the defect is usually one of ventilation.

Impending failure of respiratory mechanisms

Signs of impending failure of the respiratory mechanisms are:

(a) jerky, irregular, shallow or laboured breathing;
(b) restlessness;
(c) 'tracheal tug'—where the trachea is dragged down with every laboured breath;
(d) movement of the accessory muscles of respiration, e.g. active alae nasi;
(e) open mouth, lip-biting, anxious expression;
(f) cold extremities;
(g) sweating;
(h) drowsiness leading to unconsciousness.

As this process proceeds, cyanosis will become obvious, although carbon dioxide retention gives rise to a flushed skin. Cough and sputum may be a feature further exhausting the patient. Rales and rhonchi may be heard in the chest, and X-ray may confirm respiratory disease or fractured ribs. The blood gases will be the most important diagnostic point in the assessment. Lung function tests will probably be impossible, although a measure of the tidal volume can be made with a Wright's Respirometer (Fig. 3.10, page 81). A value below 300 ml will influence any decision to ventilate the lungs, especially if the minute volume is also low (i.e. below 4 litres). The respiratory rate will probably be raised and this will cause distress and exhaustion.

When the diagnosis of respiratory insufficiency is established, a definitive line of treatment will be commenced, and the progress followed by frequent estimation of blood gas tensions. Whatever line of treatment is taken, it must be remembered that respiratory failure is the end of an abnormal or diseased process and this must also be treated. Therefore antispasmodics, antibiotics, physiotherapy, tracheal suction, and treatment of cardiac failure may also be required.

It can be seen that mechanical ventilation (IPPV) plays an important part in the treatment of these cases, and it is here that the Intensive Care Unit has established a vital role. Whether for short term support or for long term treatment, it is safe to employ this mechanical form of ventilation under the supervision of well-trained nurses in the ICU.

Oxygen inhalation therapy

Oxygen tension in the arterial blood can be increased by raising the concentration in the inspired gases. It has now been well established that breathing 100 % oxygen even at atmospheric pressure may damage the lungs. For this reason, it is important that the inspired concentration should not be higher than necessary and should not raise the Po_2 of the arterial blood above 150 mmHg (20 kPa). For this reason accurate metering of oxygen concentration is valuable and should be varied according to the arterial Po_2. The oxygen analyser is a valuable aid to accurate oxygen therapy.

There are three groups of oxygen inhalation therapy equipment:

1 Low concentration (up to 35%)
2 High concentration (up to 60%)
3 Hyperbaric oxygen (above atmospheric pressure)

The oxygen mask is the most convenient method of adding oxygen to the inspired gases, but this is often uncomfortable for the ill patient. Ideally the mask should be light, comfortable and disposable (Fig. 3.6). It is an advantage if it is transparent, as this allows the face to be observed. It should also be inexpensive, leak-proof and have a small dead space. The alternative to a mask is an oxygen tent, but this has little place in the modern ICU since it is large and unwieldy, expensive and presents a fire hazard. In addition, an oxygen tent often produces an unsatisfactory level of oxygen therapy, as the oxygen level falls when the tent is opened for physiotherapy and other procedures. Provisions have to be made for cooling and humidity control, and oxygen tents are now restricted to children, to patients who are dyspnoeic and extremely restless, or if vomiting is a feature of the illness.

1   Low concentration oxygen masks

These are designed for controlled oxygen therapy, and employ the venturi principle to entrain air. The Ventimask (Fig. 3.6) is an example in common use and there are four different models available. The 24% (Po_2 180 mmHg or 23.9 kPa) and 28% (Po_2 210 mmHg or 27.9 kPa) models work on a 4 l/min flow of oxygen. The 35% (Po_2 270 mmHg or 35.9 kPa) model requires a higher flow of 8 l/min. (A 40% model is also available). These masks have a reliable performance and a relatively small dead space even if the oxygen supply should become inadvertently disconnected. They are, however, uncomfortable and unsuitable for the gravely ill patient with severe desaturation.

There are several other masks in use including the Edinburgh mask which will give a concentration of 33–39% oxygen with a flow of 4 l/min.

2   High concentration masks

These are the semi-rigid masks (MC and Hudson), the masks with a reservoir bag (BLB and Oxyair) and the soft plastic masks (Polymask and Pneumask). The Pneumask has rebreathing characteristics which may be undesirable. The BLB and Oxyair are uncomfortable, but the MC is well tolerated by patients, and with a flow of 3–4 l/min gives a satisfactory concentration and prevents rebreathing (Fig. 3.7). With an oxygen flow in excess of 6 l/min the inspired oxygen concentration will be reliably above 50%.

Various forms of nasal oxygen catheters are available which are easily

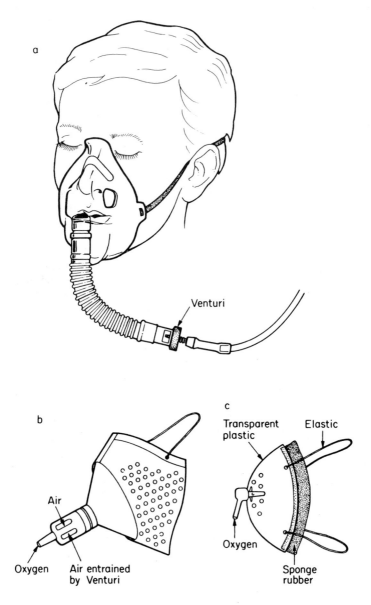

Fig. 3.6 (a) The Bard Inspiron oxygen mark
       (b) The Ventimask
       (c) The MC mask

tolerated and leave the mouth free for feeding. Intubated patients and those with a tracheostomy are best fixed to a T-piece (Fig. 3.7) with a flow of 2–3 l/min. A tracheostomy mask is also available.

This second group allows high oxygen concentrations to be administered by increasing the flow of oxygen. Where possible this should be checked with an analyser, bearing in mind that the risk of high oxygen concentrations must be set against the sequelae of acute hypoxia.

3 Hyperbaric oxygen

This produces a great increase in the dissolved oxygen in the blood. At atmospheric pressure breathing air, only 0.3 ml oxygen is in solution in each 100 ml of blood. If 100 % oxygen is breathed this is increased to approximately 2 ml. By doubling the pressure to two atmospheres the dissolved oxygen is 4 ml/100 ml and at three atmospheres 6 ml/100 ml. In theory, this amount is sufficient to supply all the oxygen required by the tissues even in the absence of red blood cells.

Although at first thought to be valuable in the treatment of a large number of conditions (e.g. burns, infections, gangrene and in combination with radiotherapy), hyperbaric oxygen is now of established value only in the treatment of some cases of carbon monoxide poisoning and gas gangrene. In carbon monoxide poisoning, it displaces carbon monoxide from carboxyhaemoglobin and, by increasing the dissolved oxygen present, prevents tissue anoxia. In gas gangrene, the activity of the organisms and the production of toxin is reduced.

Hyperbaric oxygen is normally administered in a single chamber with a sodalime carbon dioxide absorbing system. Fire is a hazard, and mechanical ventilators must be gas-driven.

Humidification

Normally, inspired air is warmed and moistened by the lining of the oral and particularly the nasal cavities. If this normal method of humidifi-

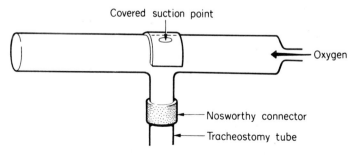

Covered suction point

Oxygen

Nosworthy connector

Tracheostomy tube

Fig. 3.7 A T-piece for oxygen administration

cation is by-passed, then artificial methods of moistening the air must be used in order to prevent drying of the mucous membranes. Dry air also depresses ciliary action so that the combined effect is crusting, ulceration and obstruction by inspissated secretions. This situation arises when the patient is intubated or when a tracheostomy has been performed. It is particularly dangerous if the patient is ventilated with dry gases, while it is not such a problem if the patient is breathing spontaneously and has a good cough reflex.

The most comfortable temperature of inspired gases appears to be about 30–36°C with an absolute humidity of approximately 30–40 mg H_2O/l of air (72–95% at 36°C). Higher temperatures can produce laryngospasm and even hyperthermia. The method of producing these conditions is by altering the properties of the inspired gases during their passage from the gas source to the patient's trachea. The methods must be suitable for both spontaneously breathing patients as well as those on ventilators. The methods available are:

1 Heat and moisture exchangers
2 Saline instillation
3 Nebulisers
4 Water-bath humidifiers

1   Heat and moisture exchangers

Appliances such as the condenser-humidifier or 'Swedish Nose' are designed to trap moisture and heat at each expiration by means of condensation on a wire gauze mesh or rolled corrugated foil. When water vapour condenses it gives up its latent heat; thus heat and moisture is added to the next inspired breath. The efficiency of these condenser humidifiers depends on the ambient temperature. They add an extra resistance to breathing, and can be a source of infection. They can give an absolute humidity of 22–24 mg/l and give an inspired temperature of 28–30°C. They are moderately comfortable and suitable, if secretions are not excessive, for patients who are improving clinically and are breathing spontaneously. Great care must be taken to ensure condenser humidifiers do not become blocked by secretions or debris.

2   Saline instillation

This may be used if other methods are not available. Physiological saline or mucolytic agents may be instilled into the endotracheal or tracheostomy tube. Excessive quantities must be avoided especially if a drip method is employed.

3   Nebulisers

These can be gas driven or mechanically driven. The gas driven nebulisers depend upon a jet of gas entraining water from a reservoir and producing a droplet mist. Sterile water must be used. The larger droplets are usually removed from the mist by a baffle. These mists can be heated or cold. The heated mists can produce humidification up to 50 mg/l whereas the cold nebulisers can produce 29 mg/l. The disadvantages of nebulisers is that the delivery tube becomes heavily laden with water, and small bore tubing may become blocked. They are difficult to sterilise and the jets may become blocked.

The mechanical nebulisers are either of the rotating disc or ultrasonic plate pattern. The ultrasonic nebuliser works on the principle that a quartz disc will oscillate if placed in an electric alternating field. This breaks up drops into a stable aerosol or mist with droplets as small as one micrometer. The disadvantage of this type of nebuliser is that these small droplets may permit large amounts of water to penetrate deeply into the lungs with consequent absorption of potentially dangerously large volumes of fluid. It is thought that infection may likewise be conveyed into the lungs. They are also expensive and have a limited life.

Nebulised substances. The nebuliser may be used to distribute droplets of bronchodilators into the lungs. It is particularly valuable in the use of such substances as salbutamol (Ventolin) which is an extremely powerful bronchodilator in the treatment of severe obstructive airway disease such as asthma. Mucolytic agents such as Airbron (acetylcysteine) can be nebulised in the same way.

4 Water-bath humidifiers

These are probably the best type of humidifier because they produce a vapour saturated at any temperature. They work by passing gas over heated water (the unheated patterns are unsatisfactory and inefficient). The aim is to produce gas saturated at a suitable temperature at the patient's end of the tubing. Condensation may occur along the length of the tubing, and attempts have been made to overcome this by lagging. These distal humidifiers should be set at about 60–70°C (which is a pasteurising temperature), to produce the correct temperature at the patient's end of the circuit. At 35°C, a humidity of approximately 40 mg/l can be produced. They are a common source of infection and should be sterilised after use and kept dry. Aqueous chlorhexidine (1 in 5000 solution) can be used in this type of humidifier to reduce the incidence of recontamination after sterilisation. Many of these devices may be sterilised by operation of an override switch which causes the water to heat up and boil. Care must be taken to ensure that this does not happen when the humidifier is connected to the breathing circuit. Although manufacturers attempt to fit fail-safe systems to prevent this happening, accidents still occur. The level of water in the humidifier must be regularly maintained. This is important when IPPV is also employed because a drop in the level of water increases the *compressible volume*, i.e. the amount of gas which can be compressed in the air-space above the water of the humidifier during the inflation phase of the ventilator, so that the volume of gas actually entering the patient's lungs is not as much as it is thought to be. In this case the tidal volume registered on the expiratory side of the circuit will be greater than that measured at the catheter mount. The difference in volume indicates the 'compressed' volume in the various lengths of tubing, in the ventilator itself and in the humidifier and represents a volume which has been delivered from the ventilator and has gone round the circuit but has *not* entered the patient's lungs.

Intermittent positive pressure ventilation (IPPV)

Indications for use

Mechanical ventilation of the lungs (IPPV) is required in cases of respiratory failure which cannot be treated satisfactorily by other means. The signs of respiratory distress which are signs of impending respiratory failure have been described on page 70, and these are warnings that respiratory support may be required. Steady deterioration shown in blood gases and the clinical condition leaves no doubt as to the course indicated, but it must be remembered that there are still some cases of mild failure that will respond to oxygen inhalation therapy with careful monitoring of blood gases, clinical state and inspired oxygen concentration.

Blood gases alone may not be helpful in borderline cases and they should be considered together with the clinical picture. However, a rising P_{CO_2} is a valuable guide especially if it should rise higher than 60 mmHg (8.0 kPa). Generally this indicates the need for IPPV, but the pre-existing medical condition must be taken into account (e.g. chronic bronchitis). Similarly, a P_{O_2} level of less than 60 mmHg breathing air indicates respiratory failure and may be a reason to commence IPPV. Clinically cyanosis, sweating, cold extremities, drowsiness, exhaustion and dyspnoea are all indications for respiratory help. In addition, the cardiovascular system may show signs of strain illustrated by tachycardia and hypotension. These may be the deciding factors in making the decision. Chest X-ray can be helpful if severe disease is demonstrated, but respiratory function tests are of little or no value.

To sum up, the decision regarding ventilation is based on many parameters, but is usually not difficult. It is safe to say that if in doubt the patient should be ventilated, as in a good unit this should not in itself constitute a hazard. One of the great advantages of IPPV is that it removes the great extra workload imposed upon a patient who is exhausted by the sheer effort of breathing.

Types of ventilator

Ventilators may be classified according to their design characteristics into astonishingly complex different types. However, the following classification is both simple and practical:

1 Pressure pre-set. In this type, the pressure is pre-set or predetermined by a 'weight on a bellows' principle (e.g. East-Radcliffe ventilator). This principle allows compensation for very small leaks in the circuit. The pressure cannot be increased unless someone alters the weight on the bellows. The disadvantage of this type of ventilator is that if the compliance of the chest falls or the airway resistance increases then the same pressure generates a smaller tidal volume.

2 Volume pre-set. Here a predetermined volume is delivered (e.g. Cape Ventilator). The volume pre-set machine is better for ventilating stiff lungs because the given volume has to be delivered no matter how great the resistance of the lungs. However, there can be no compensation for leaks because a volume greater than that which has been pre-set cannot be delivered (unless an attendant alters the controls). These machines can generate enormous pressures in the airway.

Volume, pressure and time cycling

The design characteristic of the Cape ventilator is such that it will deliver a pre-determined volume (volume pre-set). The cycling from inspiration to expiration and *vice versa* occurs after a certain time. Since the machine is mains-powered and the mechanism of bellows and valves is controlled by cams turned by an electric motor, the Cape is correctly termed a *time-cycled, electro-mechanical, volume pre-set* lung ventilator. However, these machines are simple to operate and the oxygen enrichment is easily arranged. The disadvantages of this type of ventilator are that the patient needs to be completely apnoeic, leaks may remain undetected, and the machine will continue to work if it becomes disconnected. Triggering is not possible with this type of ventilator.

Some pressure pre-set machines have the advantage that they can 'trigger' in response to a weak respiratory effort by the patient and can be used in 'weaning'. Their disadvantage is that with machines such as the Bird or Bennett the volume delivered depends on the stiffness of the lungs, because the change *from* inspiration *to* expiration depends on a certain value of pre-set pressure being reached in the patient's lungs (*pressure cycled*). If the patient's lungs are very stiff, the pre-set pressure may result in a very small volume ventilating the lungs. For this reason some gas volume measure, such as Wright's Respirometer, must be used to detect changes in compliance (p. 58). Generally, these ventilators are not good at ventilating stiff lungs or those with increased airway resistance, but they are small in size and usually inexpensive. It is often difficult to add oxygen accurately to the inspired gases unless a blender device is used.

In addition to the volume and pressure cycling, some machines may cycle according to time (*time cycling*), for example East-Radcliffe, Cape, Oxford, Nuffield 200 and Airshields ventilators. Long inflation times may help in patients with airway obstruction.

Resistance to inflation of the chest by an elastic bag depends upon the airway resistance and the elasticity of the lungs and thoracic cage. If either of these last two components is increased, the pressure required to deliver a predetermined volume of gas will be higher; the converse is also true. This concept is known as compliance and is described on page 58. A patient with asthma will have a low compliance—the increase in volume for a given increase in pressure will be low. If the compliance is changing, then the pressure required to deliver a given volume of gas will also change. Thus underventilation will result if the compliance falls. It can be seen that any pressure pre-set ventilator may require constant attention and adjustment. In low compliance states, the volume cycled or pre-set machine is preferable, where the set volume is always delivered even if the compliance changes.

Subatmospheric or 'negative' pressure. Some ventilators have provision for introducing a 'negative' phase at the end of expiration. The positive pressure in the chest during the inspiratory phase reduces venous return and may cause a reduction in cardiac output, offset by the reduction in work of breathing by the instigation of IPPV and by compensatory vasoconstriction. However, in the patient with severe cardiovascular disturbance, a fall in blood pressure may occur. The introduction of a negative pressure phase in these cases, by reducing the mean intrathoracic pressure, will diminish the effects of IPPV on the circulation. Normally, negative pressures greater than $-5\,cmH_2O\,(-0.5\,kPa)$ are not used and high 'negative' pressures may even cause 'trapping' of gas in the alveoli with consequent arterial desaturation. 'Negative' pressure is of dubious value except in patients who are hypovolaemic, where a low intrathoracic pressure is essential. A 'negative' phase can prove harmful in patients with cardiac failure as the amount of shunting (venous admixture) in the lung is increased.

End-expiratory resistance (positive end-expiratory pressure, PEEP). By sustaining the positive pressure at the end of expiration at a level of $+5$ to $+10\,cm\,H_2O\,(0.5–1.0\,kPa)$ oxygenation can be raised in patients with pulmonary atelectasis, oedema and shunts. This may be very effective if all other methods fail and can produce a dramatic improvement in the patient's oxygenation. The detrimental cardiovascular effects mentioned above must be watched for in this situation, and careful attention given to maintaining hydration and blood volume. High PEEP is used in some centres; there is a very real risk of pneumothorax developing and great care should be taken to monitor volumes and pressures in the lung. In general, a valid indication for PEEP is inability to maintain the Pa_{O_2}

above 60 mmHg (8.0 kPa) with an F_{IO_2} of 0.5.

'Sighing'. It was thought that the incorporation of a 'sigh' or deep inspiration periodically throughout mechanical ventilation would improve ventilation and diminish shunts. In practice, this is of little or no value except when small tidal volumes (e.g. 7 ml/kg) are used. It is more important to ensure adequate tidal volumes (e.g. 10–15 ml/kg body weight) rather than rely on a sigh facility.

Oxygen enrichment. This is usually required, and it is wise to raise the oxygen concentration of the inspired gases to about 30% to compensate for shunts within the lung.

Additional ventilator dead space. Some patients requiring mechanical ventilation need large tidal volumes in order to be satisfactorily controlled (see page 56). Others who are only lightly sedated may also feel uncomfortable with the tidal volumes necessary to produce acceptable blood gas levels. Excessive ventilation (i.e. tidal volumes greater than 7 ml/kg body weight) may produce a low P_{CO_2}, except in patients with a high dead-space/tidal volume ratio, and this can be rectified by the addition of 'dead space' in the form of an extra section of tubing between the Y-piece of the ventilator and the endotracheal tube connections.

Varying volume dead spaces can be tried until an acceptable P_{CO_2} is obtained. Care should be taken to check the P_{O_2} as well, as the introduction of any dead space will reduce the inspired oxygen concentration. An attractive way of achieving normocapnia with large volumes is to use the fractional rebreathing technique of the Bain co-axial breathing circuit; a normal P_{CO_2} is achieved by setting a fresh gas flow of 70 ml/kg body weight and tidal volumes of 10–15 ml/kg body weight. Lower P_{CO_2} levels are achieved simply by increasing the flow rate of fresh gas.

Connecting the ventilator

The patient either has a tracheostomy or the trachea will have been intubated. Connecting the patient to the ventilator is usually performed by the doctor, but it will be a nurse's duty in an emergency or during suction. Nosworthy or plastic ('Portex') connections are popular, and some tracheostomy tubes are manufactured with a Nosworthy fitting (Figs. 3.8 and 3.9).

Various means have been devised to prevent disconnection, and a slight twist given as the connector is pushed home helps maintain the union. Any procedure involving the ventilator/tube connection should be carried out in as aseptic a manner as possible. The connection from the ventilator is appropriately called the catheter mount (Fig. 3.9).

Management and care of patients during IPPV

Presuming that breathing is absent or controlled (page 83), the next step is to see that the ventilator is set at the correct rate and tidal volume. This

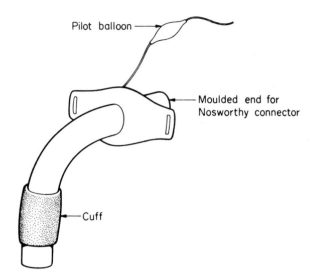

Fig. 3.8 A Portex tracheostomy tube

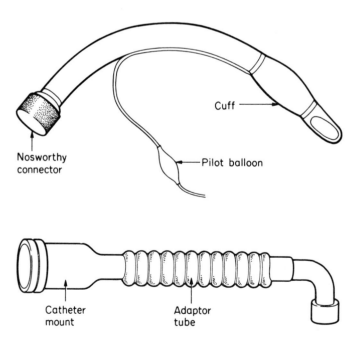

Fig. 3.9 A Magill oral endotracheal tube and catheter mount

is relatively simple in the volume-cycled machines where rate and tidal volume controls are clearly marked. In pressure-cycled machines, however, the set pressure produces a tidal volume which must be measured by a spirometer. The Radford Nomogram, which is based on surface area, is only a guide and may be of no help in severe lung disease. Usually, tidal volumes of 10–15 ml/kg are required and this volume is delivered at a rate of about 10–12 cycles/min initially, and altered if necessary on the results of the blood gas estimations. Normally, a P_{CO_2} of 30–40 mmHg (4.0–5.3 kPa) is satisfactory, but if a tidal volume which is comfortable for the patient produces a lower P_{CO_2} than desirable, an extra dead space may be added.

The inflation pressure will be shown on a gauge on the machine and this bears a relation to the compliance. A satisfactory pressure is 15–20 cmH$_2$O (1.5–2.0 kPa) or less, but this may be doubled in severe lung disease. Humidification is essential and is usually incorporated with the ventilator.

A Wright's or Draeger respirometer, or a dry displacement gas meter (Fig. 3.10) is commonly used for tidal volume measurement. The respirometers, with the exception of the dry gas meter type, may be rendered inaccurate by waterlogging if left in the circuit. Readings are therefore taken intermittently.

The composition of the gases used to ventilate the patient's lungs will depend upon the condition of the lungs and circulation. One hundred percent oxygen is undesirable and may damage the lungs. If used, it should be for the shortest possible time. Nevertheless, some added oxygen is invariably required during ventilation because of intrapulmonary

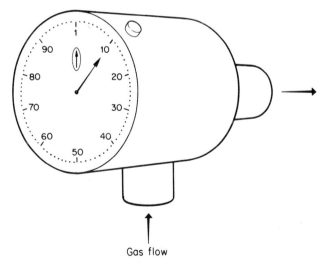

Gas flow

Fig. 3.10 Wright's Respirometer

shunting. Thirty percent is usually sufficient, and higher concentrations should be used only if indicated by unsatisfactory blood Po_2 results. A figure of 100–150 mmHg (13.3–19.5 kPa) should be the aim. Accurate metering of the concentration of oxygen in the inspired air is mandatory and inexpensive oxygen analysers are available.

Although charting of the rate, tidal volume and pressure should be carried out quarter- to half-hourly, observations of the chest movements by experienced nurses are equally important. Connections should be checked hourly and tightened where necessary.

Changes in pressure require explanation. Although changes in compliance may be the cause, they are more likely to be due to obstruction of the tube by mucus or secretions. Kinking or condensation in the ventilator tubing will require attention for the reason.

The care of the patient on a ventilator is a great responsibility. Primarily, it must be realised that the life of the patient depends upon the working of the machine. The nurse must be responsible for ensuring that the prescribed pulmonary ventilation is maintained and know how to act without delay should a machine fault develop. *The patient should be disconnected from the machine and be ventilated by hand if a serious fault develops.* A self-filling bag such as the Laerdal or the Ambu bag is a convenient way of dealing with this emergency and is easier for a nurse to manage than an anaesthetic bag-mask assembly. Other faults, such as kinking of tubes or obstruction due to secretions will be managed by the experienced nurse. Medical help will be required if unexplained changes in inflation pressure should occur. The experienced nurse will also notice when the patient requires further muscle relaxant or sedation to suppress spontaneous breathing. The general nursing care of these patients is discussed in Chapter 10.

Once the patient is established on the ventilator, arterial blood gas measurement will be required daily or more frequently.

'Fighting' the ventilator. A well-ventilated patient is one who is lying quietly and whose breathing is fully synchronised or controlled. Any loss of control will be readily spotted by the well-trained nurse who will immediately take the necessary action. She will check that the patient is not hypoxic or hypercapnic and that he is receiving the correct tidal volume. Common causes of desynchronisation from the ventilator include disconnection, leaks in the circuit, accumulation of secretions in the lungs, and obstruction or kinking of the breathing circuit, endotracheal or tracheostomy tube. The result of desynchronisation is inadequate ventilation and reduced cardiac output leading to hypoxia, which may have further disastrous effects on cardiac output and on a failing circulation. Struggling of this type also produces an increased oxygen consumption which further aggravates the situation. Anticipation of this condition is a skill gained with experience. Inadequate volume ventilation in itself may be a cause, and very often quite large tidal volumes will help to control ventilation. The over-ventilation occuring in this situation may result in a low blood P_{CO_2}. Only after all possible causes of desynchronisation have been checked should doses of sedative or muscle relaxant drugs be given.

Control of patients on ventilators

In order to obtain the full physiological advantages of automatic ventilation, the patient must be quiet and completely under the control of the ventilator. This can be attained by one of two ways:

1 Centrally depressing drugs. Many of the narcotic drugs, by their effect on the central nervous system, depress respiration sufficiently to allow control of respiration. Their analgesic effects make them particularly suitable where pain is a feature. The euphoria produced by these drugs help to produce a state of acceptance. Examples are morphine, papaveretum and phenoperidine. They should be long-acting, suitable for intravenous injection and easily reversed.

Other drugs which have a sedating effect on the CNS may also be used. Intravenous diazepam, 2.5–5.0 mg is popular. Barbiturates may also be used successfully in limited cases, as may chlorpromazine and promazine. Droperidol is used to potentiate the effect of opiates and for its neurolept and anti-emetic effect. However, droperidol should not be used on its own in awake patients as they may experience unpleasant feelings of catatonia. Nitrous oxide/oxygen mixtures such as Entonox have had some success particularly where pain is prominent. Long-term administration of nitrous oxide causes bone marrow depression and aplastic anaemia.

2 Muscle relaxants. In some cases central sedation is insufficient to affect control, hence muscle relaxants must be used. Many cases of severe left ventricular failure are not controllable on sedation alone as the drive to breathe is too strong. There are also cases where large doses of centrally depressing drugs are not desirable, for example in severe head injury or after cardiac arrest where the level of consciousness is to be assessed as soon as possible. Muscle relaxants may be used to paralyse the muscles of respiration and allow the ventilator to take over. Tubocurarine has been used extensively, but the hypotensive effect of large doses has made it undesirable particularly in cardiac patients. Gallamine triethiodide (Flaxedil) produces tachycardia and is excreted by the kidneys which may not always be functioning well. Pancuronium (Pavulon) is probably the most suitable drug. It does not produce hypotension and lasts about 40–60 minutes. Large doses have been given and appear not to be markedly affected by kidney disease. Pancuronium causes a mild tachycardia which may be a disadvantage.

Muscle relaxants produce a well-controlled patient and sedation can be added if there is fear of consciousness. This has probably been overstated and patients ventilated in the ICU on relaxants alone have not reported it as unpleasant. Many of these patients are, of course, extremely ill and are on the point of unconsciousness by virtue of their disease. The very ill and moribund can be ventilated without either relaxants or central depressants.

Muscle relaxants such as pancuronium may be given in order to initiate ventilation when the patient is intubated. Endotracheal intubation will be the first step, the patient being connected to a ventilator via the endotracheal tube. In the conscious patient, a small dose of metho-hexitone (Brietal) may be necessary in order to induce sleep.

Control of ventilation is therefore as precise as other procedures in the ICU. It is individual to each case and often involves the use of both groups of drugs. *It must never be forgotten that a paralysed patient is completely defenceless* should accidental disconnection from the ventilator occur. Muscle relaxants should not be used unless absolutely necessary.

Endotracheal intubation and tracheostomy

These procedures are carried out in the ICU for the following reasons:

1 to protect the airway from inhalation of blood, vomit, food and secretions;
2 to allow mechanical ventilation;
3 to allow suction of secretions from the trachea and bronchi;
4 to bypass obstructions in the mouth, pharynx or larynx.

In general, endotracheal intubation is carried out as an emergency procedure or if the precipitating cause is expected to exist for a short period (about one week). Tracheostomy is performed if intubation is required for a longer period of time. Occasionally tracheostomy will be performed in order to reduce dead space in severe respiratory disease, by replacing the large dead space of the oral cavity and trachea by that of a relatively small tube.

In practice all or some of these factors may co-exist. If the causative factors are capable of correction in a short period of time, endotracheal intubation with or without IPPV may suffice, until the failed system has recovered. However, if during the course of this supportive treatment it is apparent that long term treatment is necessary, then tracheostomy should be performed.

Endotracheal intubation

In general, an endotracheal tube should not be left in place for more than one week. Some units claim that with a well chosen size of plastic tube up to three weeks is safe. There is, however, evidence that such management may lead to ulceration and even tracheal stenosis. It is only in exceptional cases that the initial week should be extended, after careful visualisation of the cords and arytenoid cartilages of the larynx for damage. Although there is no good experimental evidence of the superiority of plastics over red rubber, the surface of the plastic tube is certainly smoother than the rubber.

The cuff should preferably be floppy and not small and tense. Over-inflating the cuff and placing the endotracheal tube in hot water will produce a satisfactory low pressure cuff. Various designs of purpose-designed 'low pressure' cuffs are now preferred. Improved shape of tube curvature, so that excess pressure is not exerted at the posterior part of the trachea, may reduce complications.

Nasal endotracheal tubes may be more comfortable and better tolerated by the patient. There is less kinking and no ulceration at the angles of the mouth. However, the nares may be damaged and ulcerated in the same way.

Cuff pressures should be kept as low as possible, and the volume used recorded using the same size syringe on each occasion. The cuff should be inflated until the leak is just obliterated. Any increase in the volume should be reported to the anaesthetist and an explanation sought. The presence of the endotracheal tube very soon damages the epithelium of the trachea. The practice of regular deflation of the cuff will not prevent this and, in addition, can result in periods of inadequate ventilation with the risk of aspirating secretions.

Method. Although every doctor should be capable of performing endotracheal intubation, when possible it should be carried out by an anaesthetist. In the seriously ill or moribund patient, the tube can be passed without difficulty because of the relaxed state of the jaws and larynx. The sucker should be at hand and a Portex plastic tube of the correct size (8.0–9.0 mm in the adult) passed under direct vision with a Macintosh laryngoscope. In the conscious patient a small dose of methohexitone (50–70 mg) can be used to induce sleep. This should be followed by a muscle relaxant. If ventilation is to be controlled, pancuronium 0.1 mg/kg body weight is effective for incubation and will then allow IPPV to be initiated. Facilities for inflating the lungs with oxygen must always be at hand. The cuff is then inflated until the leak is just obliterated. A nasogastric tube should be inserted into the stomach at the same time.

Complications. These can be mechanical or specific. The mechanical complications are displacement, kinking or blockage of the tube. The specific complications are hoarseness, infection, sub-glottic or glottic oedema. There may be ulceration and scarring of the larynx and trachea. Many of the complications listed in association with tracheostomy may also occur with endotracheal intubation.

Tracheostomy

Tracheostomy is associated with long-term care and carries a higher complication rate. Any patient with a tracheostomy is potentially infected and should be treated as such. A sterile suction technique will help to minimise infection. Again, plastic tubes are thought to be preferable to those made of red rubber. Silver tubes will be used in some long-term cases after the risk of aspiration has passed. These are more comfortable and can be fitted with a speaking valve.

In spite of the disadvantages of tracheostomy, it is superior to intubation for suction, more comfortable for the patient and has the advantage that the patient can speak if a valve is used.

Method. Although every doctor should be capable of performing a tracheostomy in an emergency, an experienced surgeon should be called if time permits. There is nothing worse than a badly performed tracheostomy. It is generally best to perform the operation under general anaesthesia, but local anaesthesia may be indicated. In the moribund patient no anaesthesia is required.

The skin incision should be transverse and deepened between the muscles to expose the second, third and fourth rings of the trachea. The first ring should never be incised, and care should also be taken not to perform the tracheostomy too low. Either a vertical (Fig. 3.11) or an inverted 'U' incision can be made in the front of the trachea. In the latter case, the flap ('Bjork flap') can be sewn to the deep fascia or skin. This flap of cartilage provides support below the tracheostomy tube and very much facilitates the correct introduction of a replacement tube. The largest size tube to make a snug fit should be inserted and fastened with tapes. The

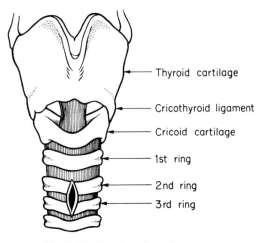

Fig. 3.11 The site of tracheostomy

average female patient takes a size of 32–36 FG* and the male 36–42 FG. These tubes have no inner tube and therefore may need to be changed twice weekly. Double tubes made of silastic are too expensive for routine use. The cuff pressure should be recorded as with endotracheal tubes and suction performed hourly (page 186). If obstruction occurs it will result in atelectasis and hypoxia. Artificially 'coughing' the patient may help to remove secretions. Physiotherapy will be required, together with turning.

Cricothyrotomy rather than tracheostomy is becoming preferred in some Intensive Care Units. It is believed that cricothyrotomy (where the tube is inserted through an incision made in the membrane between the cricoid and thyroid cartilages) is less likely to be associated with airway stenosis than tracheostomy.

Complications. These are numerous but, with the exception of mechanical malpositioning and disconnection, relatively uncommon. Obstruction has been mentioned and will be remedied by changing the tube. The more serious complications are infection (*Pseudomonas, Pyocyaneas, Streptococcus,* etc.), ulceration, stenosis, tracheal dilation and collapse, fistula, haemorrhage, surgical emphysema and disturbances of swallowing. Pressure erosion of the tracheal wall and fatal haemorrhage from neck vessels have been reported.

'Weaning' from the ventilator

This requires skill in observation, patience, and a compassionate attendant. Signs that a patient is ready to come off the ventilator will be a clear chest X-ray, satisfactory blood gases on minimal enrichment with oxygen, satisfactory cardiovascular, renal and cerebral state and a favourable clinical impression. Having ensured that the patient is not under the influence of either muscle relaxants or central sedation, the ventilator can be either used as an assister or 'trigger' or, if the patient is fit enough, dispensed with altogether. If triggering with the Bird Ventilator, the action is explained to the patient and the setting is one requiring minimal effort. If small ineffective breaths are taken, the triggering effort should be increased so that the machine will only assist reasonably adequate breaths. If the patient can manage this technique, it is immediately apparent and his general condition is then observed for tachycardia, sweating or cyanosis.

Usually, if a patient is fit enough to come off the ventilator this can be achieved in one step by discontinuing the use of the ventilator altogether. Added oxygen can be given through a T-piece and the patient's condition watched carefully for deterioration. Any sign of cyanosis, sweating, tachypnoea or fall in blood pressure is a sign to put the patient back on the ventilator. Traditional practice is to start with 10–15 minute periods off

* FG, French gauge.

the ventilator each hour during the day, using the ventilator at night. This can be gradually increased until the patient is off the ventilator all day and then finally off both day and night. Added oxygen can be gradually reduced and finally discontinued if the blood gases allowed. In some patients, this may be a prolonged process while others can be taken off in one step. During this time, physiotherapy and suction are vital.

Another and more popular method of weaning patients from ventilator therapy is to introduce *intermittent mandatory ventilation* (IMV). This allows the patient to breathe spontaneously whenever he likes through the IMV valve, and hence to bypass the ventilator, while the 'controlled' breaths delivered from the ventilator are set to come in at a few times a minute. The number of controlled breaths is progressively reduced over a period of time until the whole of the patient's ventilation is made up of satisfactory spontaneous breaths. Another method of weaning is called *mandatory minute ventilation* (MMV), where the *minute volume* determined is made up of a combination of spontaneous breaths taken by the patient and controlled 'mandatory' breaths delivered from the ventilator. An endotracheal tube should be removed only when it is certain that the use of ventilation is no longer required. The pharynx and trachea must be given a final aspiration followed by several deep breaths delivered from an inflating bag to re-expand any atelectatic areas of lung, before extubation. A useful way to extubate patients is to apply a very large tidal volume just at the moment the cuff is deflated and the tube is removed. A suction catheter held in the posterior part of the pharynx during this manoeuvre will aspirate the mucus which has accumulated between the vocal cords and the upper border of the cuff, and which is literally blown out by this artificial cough during the extubation.

In spontaneous respiration the tracheostomy tube can be used with the cuff deflated if the swallowing reflexes are functioning satisfactorily. A silver tracheostomy tube may be used with a speaking valve to allow suction if necessary. When the tracheostomy is no longer required, the tube is removed and a loose dressing applied to the cleaned tracheostome. Healing is spontaneous.

Sterilisation of ventilators

As patients on ventilators are prone to infection, ventilators should ideally be changed often. The tubing and breathing circuit should certainly be changed at least every 24 hours. Ventilators are a source of cross-infection if not adequately sterilised, and facilities for this must be freely available. Humidifiers must be stored dry and must be sterilised together with tubing. Tubing can be autoclaved or sterilised by chemical means and the humidifiers washed out with 1 % Hycolin or other suitable disinfectant. Sterile distilled water must always be used for humidification. Mineral deposits from tap water may clog and damage the thermostat mechanisms. This could cause a thermostat failure, resulting in a burned patient.

Various methods have been employed to sterilise the ventilator itself, and one of the most effective is to use a mist of 70 % ethanol or isopropyl alcohol produced by an ultrasonic nebuliser. Because this is an explosive suspension, the ventilator must first be filled with nitrogen which is run in for two minutes. This flushes out in the air and renders the procedure safe because nitrogen is an inert gas. The ventilator is converted into a closed circuit by attaching a 2 litre bag to the Y-piece and connecting the expiratory port to the room air inlet. The ventilator is then allowed to cycle for 2–3 hours while the nebulised isopropyl alcohol in nitrogen is introduced into the circuit via the supplementary oxygen inlet.

The isopropyl alcohol is run from a standard infusion set on to the vibrating plate at a rate of 15–20 drops per minute. This produces an efficient mist with particle size below 1 μm. The ventilator is then operated in clean air for about one hour in order to clear out all isopropyl alcohol before use. A shorter period, preferably not less than 20 minutes, may have to be accepted to meet the needs of the unit.

Sterilisation with ethylene oxide (10 % in carbon dioxide to reduce the risk of explosion) is expensive and requires special equipment and facilities for exhausting the gas through water. If the whole machine is to be sterilised, a special chamber or a plastic bag is required. Hydrogen peroxide can also be nebulised using the ultrasonic nebuliser, but it is an irritant to the skin and may damage parts of the ventilator. Formaldehyde vapour can be used for the internal and external parts of the ventilator, preferably in a specially designed chamber. The vapour is allowed to circulate through the machine while it is running as a closed system. Excess formaldehyde vapour can be neutralised with ammonia at the end of the sterilising process. However, the ventilator should then be run using clean air to remove all residual traces of any formaldehyde or ammonia vapour. The whole process takes 24 hours. Failure to eliminate all traces of these agents can lead to dangerous bronchospasm in the next patient to be connected to the ventilator.

Pressure-cycled machines such as the Bird are easier to sterilise than the bellows type described above. The outlet and inlet ports may be wiped with Hycolin or 5 % Milton. The plastic hoses can be soaked in Milton or 0.5 % chlorhexidine in spirit. Autoclavable or disposable hoses can be fitted. The exterior of any ventilator can be cleaned with any effective antiseptic such as Hycolin, Milton or chlorhexidine.

Sterilisation of ventilators is best achieved with completely removable patient circuits and bellows units so that the whole of the breathing system can be autoclaved. Where possible, air taken into the ventilator should be filtered. Bacterial filters on the inspiratory and expiratory parts have been used; a careful watch must be kept that these do not become clogged and so obstruct expiration. Some expiratory filters are heated by an electrical circuit to prevent condensation and so the risk of increased resistance to breathing. Checks are necessary to ensure that the temperature of these units is properly controlled.

Whenever a ventilator, valves or patient tubing are being reassembled after sterilisation, there is always the possibility of a misassembly. Although manufacturers try to make safeguards by the use of special locating pins, for instance, a misassembly occurs from time to time and there is a fatality due to failure to test the reassembled machine. The same applies to humidifiers and the way they are connected to the breathing circuit of the ventilator.

Respiratory monitoring

The best method of monitoring respiration is by trained observation. The intensive care nurse needs to learn to recognise adequate ventilation by watching the movement of the chest. This should be an even expansion, and synchronous with the ventilator if the breathing is controlled. It should not be jerky, fast or noisy. Respiratory rate and inflation pressure should be charted quarter-hourly. Any changes should be noted and acted upon.

More sophisticated methods of monitoring respiration have not been entirely satisfactory. However, measurement of tidal volume or the amount exhaled at each breath may be estimated by the use of a well-fitting face mask and the Wright's Respirometer. A more accurate measurement is possible if an endotracheal tube is in place. Mechanical ventilators are usually equipped with a respirometer in the circuit so that frequent measurements can be made and recorded at least quarter- to half-hourly. It should be realised that with some ventilators a reading on the respirometer does not necessarily mean that the patient is being ventilated with that volume. In other words, other respiratory observations are required at the same time. The minute volume can be calculated by multiplying the tidal volume by the respiratory rate. The only measurements of tidal or minute volume which have any meaning are *expired* values. No reliance should be put on inspired values except to note that if there is a substantial difference from the expired values, there is a leak somewhere in the circuit.

More complex equipment can be used to measure gas flow. The pneumatachograph will do this but requires calibration as well as technical assistance. Blood gas measurements will assess the efficiency of respiration in oxygenation and removing carbon dioxide.

Indirect measurement of the thoracic cage movements can be made by micro-switches attached to strings around the chest wall. Interference and delay in picking up respiratory failure makes this method unreliable. This also applies to strain gauges around the thorax. Other methods include impedance changes, auditory signals and diaphragm electromyography. All these are difficult measurements to stablise and are as yet unreliable. Air displacement measurements using thermistors to measure temperature changes in the oral or nasal cavities seem to be more satisfactory than methods using the detection of oxygen and carbon dioxide in the expired gases.

Respiratory function tests

Clinical impressions are not always sufficient in the diagnosis of respiratory failure. Tests of respiratory function may be of considerable help in deciding those cases which are borderline. They may, however, be difficult to perform in the severely ill patient, and often blood gas values will have to be the main guide. Simple tests of respiratory function are:

1 *Tidal volume.* This can easily be measured at the bedside using the Wright's Respirometer (normal 350–500 ml).

2 *Minute volume.* This can also be measured with the same instrument over an accurately-timed minute (normal 4–6 litres).

3 *Peak Flow.* This can be measured using a Peak Flow meter (normal expiratory 500 l/min).

4 *Forced Expiratory Volume.* This is a more difficult test and is usually measured as $FEV_{1.0}$ (i.e. the volume forcibly expired in one second), which should be 75% or more of the vital capacity.

These tests assess the volumes of the respiratory compartments and detect evidence of airway obstruction. They can be carried out at the bedside and, taken in conjunction with clinical impressions, can form the basis for decisions regarding artificial ventilation requirements. Usually this decision can be made on the clinical picture and confirmed by blood gases. In practice, their usefulness is limited and the tidal volume is all that the sick patient can manage. Other more sophisticated measurements normally have a limited place in the ICU; these include measurements of pressure, flow and volume during the breathing cycle, with computation of airway resistance and compliance.

Acid-base and blood gas measurements

This service must be available on a 24 hour basis. Without it, patients can neither be properly assessed nor their progress followed. Clinical impressions can often be misleading, and the blood gas results may be the deciding factor in the decision regarding ventilation.

There are three main measurements to be made from a sample of blood—the acidity of the blood, the level of oxygenation and the tension of the carbon dioxide.

The acidity or pH of the sample may be measured directly with a pH electrode. The tension of carbon dioxide (Pco_2) may vary according to this, as we have seen that a rise in blood P_{CO_2} will produce a *respiratory acidosis* with a fall in pH. A fall in P_{CO_2} will produce a *respiratory alkalosis* and the opposite effect on the pH. P_{CO_2} changes are not the only cause of pH changes. The acidosis may be due to accumulation of metabolic acid substances and the sample will show a decrease in bicarbonate buffer in the blood. Under these circumstances, the P_{CO_2} may be normal. The latter is known as a *metabolic acidosis*.

The P_{CO_2} is measured directly using the Severinghaus or similar electrode. Another method is to derive the P_{CO_2} using the Astrup method. This involves the measurement of three pH values using the pH electrode. From the Siggaard-Andersen curve nomogram, the following results are obtainable: pH, P_{CO_2}, standard bicarbonate, actual bicarbonate, buffer base and base excess. The respiratory and metabolic components of the acid-base disturbance can be interpreted from these results. Modern blood gas machines are virtually automatic with printing of results on a card. The introduction of unheparinised blood into such a machine will clog and seriously damage the system.

The P_{CO_2} can also be estimated from the end-tidal carbon dioxide concentration using an infra-red analyser. The method is not very accurate in the presence of lung disease, and the rebreathing method may be preferable. In the latter technique analysis of an equilibrated gas sample is made following rebreathing. This gives a figure for the mixed venous P_{CO_2}. Arterial P_{CO_2} is usually taken as 6 mmHg lower. This method can even be used on patients who are being ventilated.

Measurements of the oxygen saturation of haemoglobin in the blood can be made using an oximeter. Of greater value is the direct measurement of P_{O_2} using a polarographic oxygen electrode. It can be seen from the oxygen dissociation curve that large changes in P_{O_2} may alter the saturation by only a small amount. Ear lobe oximeters use spectrophotometric methods, but the results are affected by the circulation and the degree of vasodilatation.

When assessing lung function, it is always important to know the oxygen concentration in the inspired gases. This can be simply measured by a paramagnetic oxygen analyser, a fuel cell analyser or a fast response oxygen electrode.

Methods of taking arterial samples. Arterial samples are preferred, except in small children where arterialised venous or capillary blood can be used. The sample is usually taken from the brachial artery or the radial artery. The sample is taken into a heparinised 5 ml syringe through a 23–25 gauge needle. 0.5 ml (1000 units/ml) of heparin is taken into the syringe to wet the surface and then ejected. This leaves a small volume in the hub which is enough to heparinise the sample. 2–3 ml of blood is taken from the artery and care is taken to exclude air. The sample is sealed off by a cap or blind needle hub and the syringe rotated quickly between the palms of the hands to promote mixing. Firm pressure applied immediately to the puncture site for at least 5 minutes will prevent haematoma formation. If analysis is to be delayed beyond 20 minutes the sample should be stored in a Thermos flask containing a mixture of ice and water; at $0°C$ metabolism of the blood is greatly reduced and errors in the subsequent analyses for blood gases will be minimised.

Management of acidosis

An acid pH (lower than 7.36) can be of respiratory (see page 62) or metabolic origin. Respiratory acidosis can be diagnosed from a knowledge of the patient's history, clinical condition and the blood gas analysis, which will show a raised P_{CO_2}. This can usually be corrected by increasing the minute volume ventilation and will probably require IPPV. If the patient is already on a ventilator the rate or tidal volume may need to be increased. Care should be taken never to reduce the P_{CO_2} suddenly from a high value to a much lower value as this may precipitate two problems; firstly cardiac dysrhythmias may develop, and secondly the circulation, which may have been stimulated by the effect of a raised P_{CO_2} on cardiac output, may become suddenly depressed. The management of acid-base imbalance is described on page 37.

Chest injuries

Chest injuries are common as a result of motor traffic accidents. They are the cause of approximately one-quarter of the deaths from road accidents and may be associated with haemorrhage and damage to lung tissue. Mechanical instability results when part of the chest wall is unstable or 'flail'. Flail segments may also be produced by over-enthusiastic cardiac massage. These will usually involve a central segment in which the sternum is unsupported. The flail segment of the chest wall is sucked in during inspiration so making it impossible for the underlying lung to receive adequate ventilation. This is the so-called *paradoxical respiration*. The result is alveolar hypoventilation with hypoxaemia and hypercapnia, an increased work of breathing and an increase in atelectasis and intrapulmonary shunting. This is because the FRC (page 57) of the lung is reduced and the flailing part of the chest wall compresses the lung. In addition, the patient will be unable to cough and remove secretions because of pain. This further aggravates a serious situation. The patient shows tachypnoea, sweating and restlessness. Other injuries may also be present such as ruptured spleen and abdominal injuries. Signs of haemorrhage may require urgent operation.

All but the mildest cases of flail chest are treated by tracheostomy and IPPV. Even a healthy young adult cannot tolerate double fractures involving four ribs or more. Some centres prefer to control the flail segment by internal or external fixation of the thoracic cage but, except in the case of 'flail sternum', fixation is usually less satisfactory than IPPV. In the emergency situation, IPPV should be started without delay via an endotracheal tube. If the patient with severe paradoxical respiration is to survive, ventilation must be instituted early, during the initial management. Added oxygen will almost certainly be required as there will be some degree of intrapulmonary shunting. The necessary concentration should be carefully measured and the arterial Po_2 not allowed to rise above 150 mmHg (19.5 kPa). Antibiotic cover may be required and any pneumothorax should be treated by underwater drainage. Suction and physiotherapy are vital in order to remove secretions. It is important to maintain good nutrition in these patients. Mechanical ventilation is usually required for at least three weeks. Any marked degree of paradoxical respiration at this stage is an indication that a further period of ventilation is required. When the patient is eventually weaned from the ventilator, only the mildest degree of paradox is acceptable and then only if the blood gases are satisfactory and the patient is clinically able to manage satisfactorily. Analgesics will have been cut down in the last days prior to weaning.

Chest injuries may result in rupture of the trachea, bronchi or oesophagus. Bronchopleural fistula and other complications such as tension pneumothorax and mediastinal and subcutaneous emphysema can develop. Severe contusion of the lungs can be produced by some chest injuries with little to see in the way of outward damage. The injury to the lung caused by a sudden deceleration force leads to widespread patchy damage. The chest X-ray may show little change at first but hypoxaemia develops and the X-ray shows the changes associated with widespread pulmonary oedema. These cases can be among the most difficult to treat and the absence of fractured ribs or other injuries often leads to false optimism.

The condition just described is one of the many and varied causes of 'shock lung'. This is a rather unfortunate term as it may exist in a patient who has not suffered a cardiovascular insult. The causes of 'shock lung' include bronchospasm, fat embolism, cardiac failure, pulmonary oedema, overtransfusion, oxygen toxicity, aspiration pneumonitis, depletion of pulmonary surfactant and disseminated intravascular coagulation (page 166). The syndrome usually presents 24–48 hours after the initiating event. In extreme cases hypoxaemia is severe despite all measures and the lung appears opaque on X-ray (known as a 'white out' from the widespread opacity seen in the lung fields on the X-ray film).

Some patients with damaged lungs may demonstrate the recently recognised phenomenon of hyperoxic shunt. As the inspired oxygen concentration is increased above about 40%, more of the pulmonary blood flow passes through channels which bypass ventilated alveoli. Thus, paradoxically, increasing the inspired oxygen concentration in some patients may be associated with an increase in venous admixture (shunt) and hence a reduction in arterial oxygenation. Conversely, it is always worth finding out whether a high inspired oxygen concentration (above 40%) is really so necessary, as a reduction in the concentration may lead to an actual improvement in the patient's arterial oxygenation.

Physiotherapy

The physiotherapist should be a part of the intensive care team and a physiotherapy service should always be available. Patients on ventilators may require physiotherapy every two or three hours and this can be carried out with the assistance of the anaesthetist or nurse who will ventilate the patient's lungs by hand during the treatment. Manual ventilation can also be used to produce an artifical cough that will help to clear secretions. The unconscious patient will be turned hourly, and the head of the bed can be lowered while percussion and shaking of the lung bases is carried out after turning. This should be synchronous with expiration and, after some minutes of therapy, suction performed. If this does not disturb the patient too much, the procedure can be repeated on the other side. During physiotherapy, the patient's condition should be carefully watched; marked alteration in pulse or colour is a sign that the treatment should be discontinued. In patients with fractured ribs or after thoracotomy, analgesics should be given in suffcient time to take effect before treatment starts.

The conscious patient will be able to co-operate with the above procedures. Bronchodilators may be combined with physiotherapy. Breathing exercises and physiotherapy should be continued when mechanical ventilation is discontinued. Intensive physiotherapy will re-expand collapsed segments of lung and, by draining secretions, prevent atelectasis occurring. Patients on ventilators and those breathing relatively dry gases have a marked decrease in ciliary action in the bronchial tree and require help to clear normal secretions and abnormal secretions produced by infection. Pressure breathing with a Bird ventilator is a useful aid. in physiotherapy.

Liquefaction of secretions

The thick sticky secretions can be thinned by mucolytic drugs such as acetylcysteine (Airbron). This can be instilled into the trachea or placed in the humidifier. Bromhexine (Bisolvon) has a mucolytic action and will also increase the amount of sputum produced but will lower the viscosity. The drug can be taken orally.

Paediatric considerations

The neonate and infant cannot be considered as a miniature adult. For this reason, paediatricians are naturally reluctant to treat their patients in the general intensive care ward. Prevention of cross-infection is of paramount importance.

Because of the technical problems associated witĥ the size and situation of the trachea, endotracheal intubation has been favoured as an alternative to tracheostomy. It may be conveniently performed through the nose using a Jackson Rees nasal tube (Fig. 3.12) which may be left in place for periods well in excess of the usual one week. There are, however, problems associated with fixation and suction; also subglottic stenosis has been known to occur. For this reason, some units still prefer to use tracheostomy if more than a week of intubation will be required. When an endotracheal tube is used in an infant or small child there must always be a slight leak of air around the tube. If there is not, then the tube is too large and damage to the larynx at the cricoid will occur; a change to the smaller tube should be made. A snugly fitting non-cuffed tracheostomy tube enables IPPV to be performed with much reduced risk of tracheal damage. Scrupulous care in performing the tracheostomy and aftercare minimises some of the complications which are similar to those occurring in the adult. Safe humidification is a problem and hot water humidifiers are probably best as long as great care is taken with temperature control. Maintaining a temperature of 60–70°C may prove dangerous following disconnection for suction. Scalding may be produced when the ventilator is reconnected. Suction should be performed without disconnecting the ventilator. There is a smaller choice of lung ventilators for infants and children than for adults. Popular ventilators for infants or small children in the UK are the Draeger Babylog, Siemens Servoventilator, Engstrom,

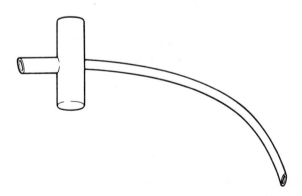

Fig. 3.12 A paediatric nasotracheal tube for long-term intubation

Erica Loosco Amsterdam, Sheffield-East, Bear and some versions of the Bennett Ventilator. Ventilation may be established with the aid of ventilation nomograms and adjusted according to blood gas analysis. Samples should preferably be taken from an artery or from a catheter in the umbilical artery. Unfortunately, heel prick samples may give unreliable results.

4

The Renal System

Physiological considerations

The kidneys have excretory, metabolic and hormonal functions (Table 4.1). Some of these functions are unique to the kidneys, while others are shared by other organs, such as the liver, which can compensate for the kidneys at least in the short term. For example, the normal liver contains sufficient vitamin D to compensate for several weeks for the absence of the vitamin newly modified by the kidneys. Abnormalities of calcium metabolism due to low vitamin D levels are therefore not clinically apparent during acute renal failure. This particular renal function can therefore be ignored in the short term and is not a problem in the Intensive Care Unit.

The unique functions of the kidneys, not shared by other organs, are the excretion of four main classes of substances—excess water, acid (hydrogen ion), electrolyte (sodium, potassium), and nitrogenous waste products derived from protein catabolism. Each of the four functions must be considered separately to understand the management of the patient with renal failure.

Renal failure is said to be *acute* when all four functions cease simultaneously and completely. *Chronic* renal failure develops over months or years, and loss of each of the four functions is incomplete. It varies from one patient to another, so that while nearly all patients have difficulty in excreting protein waste products, some have no trouble excreting water while others develop oedema. Patients suffering from

Table 4.1 Kidney functions

Excretion of:
  excess water
  excess H^+
  excess electrolyte
  excess nitrogen waste products
  drugs, chemical, hormones
Formation of:
  erythropoietin
  vitamin D
  renin
Metabolism of:
  drugs
  chemicals
  hormones

---

chronic renal failure are much more likely to develop sudden complete renal failure when subjected to stress such as blood loss. For this reason they may require admission to the ICU. Acute renal failure occurring in such patients has a worse prognosis than in a patient with previously healthy kidneys. Uncomplicated chronic renal failure is not treated in the ICU.

Acute renal failure (acute tubular necrosis, ATN)

The most striking feature of this syndrome is the complete, or almost complete, suppression of urine secretion. The daily urine volume is less that 250 ml and although it may be discoloured and appear concentrated, it contains only small amounts of the normal urinary solutes. Thus, the specific gravity of the urine is low.

The onset of ATN is characteristically sudden, usually following a period of hypotension of at least an hour, combined with at least one other factor. The associated factors commonly include sodium depletion (from vomiting, blood or plasma loss, for example), infection (especially gram-negative septicaemia), jaundice (especially obstructive jaundice), and pregnancy (especially when complicated by pre-eclampsia).

Some of these factors occur together and this seems to make renal injury more likely. Time also plays an important part, so that the prompt correction of abnormalities as they occur can often prevent the onset of ATN. Thus, in battle trauma, which is a potent cause of ATN because of a combination of blood loss and heavy bacterial soiling, it has been shown that restoration of the blood volume with plasma, if done within three hours of the original injury, will at least halve the incidence of ATN, while transfusion delayed for five hours will not reduce the incidence significantly.

Many toxic materials when eaten or injected are capable of causing ATN. They include frank poisons such as carbon tetrachloride, and drugs such as neomycin, gentamicin and tetracycline.

In all patients, the presence of pre-existing renal disease, even if asymptomatic, greatly increases the chances of developing ATN.

Acute renal failure does not cause pain in the kidneys or bladder when it has developed, and a period of a day or more can elapse before it is apparent that the patient is failing to pass urine. In this period he may continue to eat and drink, or perhaps be given intravenous fluids, so that he becomes overloaded with substances which he cannot now excrete. The symptoms experienced can be separated into four main groups to match the four main renal functions.

1   Water

Water is taken into the body by drinking, in solid food (most of which is at least 50 % water) and by the metabolism of carbohydrate, which provides about 200 ml in 24 hours. The amount of water derived from liquid and solid food varies from one individual to another, and mainly depends on the amount of fluid taken. Average amounts are about 1.5–2 litres taken as fluids, and about 400 ml derived from solid food. The total averages about 2–2.5 litres per 24 hours, which is greatly in excess of requirement. The surplus is excreted as dilute urine.

When smaller amounts of fluid are taken the urine volume falls. Even when no oral fluids are taken, enough water is derived from solid food and metabolic water to enable normal kidneys to excrete the daily load of waste products. These may be dissolved in as little as 400 ml of water to produce a maximally concentrated urine. Additionally, some water is lost as vapour in the breath (about 200 ml per 24 hours) and some in the sweat. The amount lost in the sweat depends on the patient's temperature, the surrounding air temperature, and the amount of muscular work undertaken. It can amount to 10–12 litres per day in hot dry climates. In the controlled environment of the ICU the estimate is about 300 ml per 24 hours for an apyrexial adult.

Thus the total unavoidable loss is about 750 ml per 24 hours, more or less being allowed depending on the size of the patient or the presence of pyrexia. In acute renal failure with no urine output the unavoidable loss is about 500 ml per day. Once the patient is normally hydrated, the total daily input of fluid must not exceed this amount. Obviously allowances must be made for losses of water in vomit, diarrhoea stool, exudation from wounds and burns, losses from surgical drains, seepage of cerebrospinal fluid, and equivalent amounts added to the daily fluid ration to maintain correct balance.

An assessment of the water balance of all patients with acute renal failure must be made at twice-daily intervals, when the input and output totals are checked and the fluid input for the next 12 hours is prescribed. Daily weight is a most useful running check on fluid balance charts, and some ICUs are provided with continuous weighing beds for this purpose.

It should be remembered when examining fluid balance charts over a period of days that most acute renal failure patients (indeed most patients nursed in an ICU) are in a catabolic state and will lose flesh at the rate of about 0.5 kg per day. Hypercatabolic patients with burns and crush injuries will lose weight even faster, perhaps 1–1.5 kg per day for several days, and this loss will be revealed by the daily weighing charts. Attempts to keep the weight steady by transfusing intravenous fluids will result in over-hydration of the patient.

In assessing the state of hydration the most important factor is the size of the intravascular volume. Fluid which is outside the circulation (such as ascites or peripheral oedema) may be unsightly, but it is not dangerous as long as it stays where it is. Oedema matters most when it is present in the lungs, where it impairs gas exchange and predisposes to infection, but it can be temporarily ignored in most other sites. Increasing the intravascular volume causes a rise in the central venous pressure (CVP, page 9) and when this exceeds 15 cmH$_2$O (1.5 kPa) pulmonary oedema is likely to occur. Intravenous infusions must be limited to amounts which maintain the CVP below this level. In practice a CVP of around 10 cmH$_2$O (1.0 kPa) provides a satisfactory cardiac output without danger of pulmonary oedema.

On the other hand, there is nothing to be gained by keeping the CVP at abnormally low levels. Such a policy, which implies maintaining a low circulating blood volume, can only make matters worse by ensuring a sub-optimal circulation. Intravenous fluid should be given until the CVP is at the optimum level, even if doing so causes oedema of the legs and sacrum. When this course of action is taken the CVP must be monitored hourly as occasionally, for reasons unknown, oedema fluid may become mobilised and transferred back to the intravascular space, causing a sudden rise in CVP over a matter of hours. Acute, possibly fatal, pulmonary oedema then ensues. If this should happen, fluids must be removed immediately from the circulation to reduce the CVP. Peritoneal dialysis or haemodialysis is used for this purpose. The techniques will be discussed separately.

2 Sodium and potassium

Both these electrolytes are present in all foodstuffs of animal or vegetable origin—that is to say in all food that has not been specially purified. Both are consumed in considerable excess and the unrequired surplus is excreted mainly by the kidneys. The only other normal route of excretion is the sweat, whose concentration of electrolytes is approximately half that of the plasma; significant quantities can be lost only if sweating is profuse and prolonged.

Although there is no other normal route for sodium and potassium loss, very large amounts of sodium can be lost by vomiting or by continuous gastric aspiration. Furthermore, very significant quantities of potassium can be lost from the lower intestinal tract in diarrhoea fluid, causing hypokalaemia.

If the daily intake of sodium and potassium falls below the amount lost in the sweat, as in a patient unable to absorb food, the normal kidney excretes none at all in the urine, although a diseased kidney may continue to do so. Of course, in order to perform its role in regulating electrolyte excretion, the kidney requires a normal circulation and, if the cardiac output is low, it may conserve sodium and water when it should be excreting them, so that oedema results. When this happens, the situation can be improved either by improving the cardiac output (e.g. by converting a dysrhythmia to sinus rhythm) or by giving a diuretic drug such as frusemide. Diuretics work on the kidneys by preventing the conservation of sodium, which then appears in the urine. Sodium loss is accompanied by water loss and the patient's oedema then diminishes—

always provided that he is prevented from replenishing the loss by eliminating salt from his diet and therapy.

Hyponatraemia is almost always dilutional in origin, and the result of replacing sodium-rich losses (e.g. by gastric aspiration) with sodium-poor intravenous fluids such as 5 % dextrose. It is seldom a serious problem and can be quickly corrected by giving hypertonic saline (5 % saline) in calculated amounts. Hyponatraemia is also present in Addison's disease (page 121), where it is the cause of all the symptoms, and in the rare instances of *salt-losing nephritis* when the kidneys continue to lose salt in the urine even when the serum sodium is low. Both these conditions can be corrected by giving extra salt.

Potassium retention (hyperkalaemia) is a more serious problem than sodium retention because small excess amounts of potassium can prove fatal by causing cardiac dysrhythmias (page 16). Although, rarely, potassium-losing states occur in renal disease, potassium retention is very much more common and most patients with acute or chronic renal failure have serum potassium levels higher than normal in spite of eating a low potassium diet. In acute renal failure potassium excretion virtually ceases, and potassium intake must be reduced or stopped. Because very small amounts of potassium can greatly elevate the serum potassium all possible sources, including drugs and intravenous injections, must be checked for their potassium content and alternatives used. Frequent checking of the serum potassium, at least at daily intervals, is the only safe way of monitoring. It is not safe to rely on electrocardiographic changes such as peaking of the T waves as an early warning of hyperkalaemia. The characteristic changes may be seen only immediately before a fatal dysrhythmia, and sometimes they do not occur at all.

Even in the absence of dietary potassium, the serum potassium will continue to rise in renal failure patients, especially those with a poor circulation or increased metabolic rate. This is because muscle and tissue breakdown continues in these catabolic patients, releasing quantities of intracellular potassium into the circulation. In the absence of the normal means of excreting such a load, a rise in the serum potassium is inevitable.

Potassium can be slowly extracted from such a patient by giving an ion exchange resin orally or by enema. These substances take up potassium from the patient's colon in exchange for sodium or calcium. The potassium, bound to the resin, is then safely passed into the faeces. The usual method is Resonium A, 15–20 g three or four times per day, which takes up potassium in exchange for sodium. When it is not desired to give the patient more sodium Zeocarb may be used, similarly exchanging for calcium, but this method is much more expensive. Obviously, ion exchange resins are useless in the presence of paralytic ileus and are ineffective in a patient afflicted by vomiting.

A short-term reduction in the serum potassium of about 2 mmol/l can be obtained by injecting intravenously 20 units of soluble insulin with 50 g glucose. This manoeuvre drives back into cells some of the potassium which has leaked out. The effect lasts for two or three hours and the dose can be repeated. This method is particularly useful when preparing a patient for a long journey to a dialysis centre, or as an adjunct to ion exchange resin treatment when waiting for the resin to act. It is not a feasible method for continuous control of the serum potassium.

In the last resort, haemodialysis or peritoneal dialysis may be necessary to remove the excess potassium from the hyperkalaemic patient with renal failure (page 106).

3   Acid

The *long-term* regulation of plasma pH is accomplished by excretion by the kidneys of ingested acids and of fixed acids formed from metabolism. In the *short-term*, the plasma pH is kept at 7.35–7.45 by the neutralisation or buffering of new acid by bicarbonate, haemoglobin and phosphate buffers. These buffer systems prevent the existence of free hydrogen ion in the plasma, first combining it with bicarbonate ion to form carbonic acid, which is then broken down to carbon dioxide and water, the carbon dioxide being eliminated by respiration (page 56). Obviously, the kidneys play no part in this process. However, normal metabolism also creates fixed acids such as lactic acid which cannot be eliminated in this way. The total amount of fixed acid in the normal individual amounts to about 70 mmol H^+ per day. If allowed to accumulate, this would progressively occupy the buffer systems, leading to a downward drift of pH. When the figure of 7.35 has been passed, the patient is said to be acidotic and begins to show symptoms of acidosis. The kidneys must, therefore, excrete this acid load.

Although normal kidneys are easily capable of excreting the 70–100 mmol of acid which is daily presented to them, they cannot cope with a sudden large increase in the amount of acid to be excreted, whether it is the result of abnormal metabolism (as in diabetic pre-coma) or because of an increased intake of fixed acid via the intestine, such as occurs in an overdose of aspirin (acetylsalicylic acid). In these circumstances the pH of the plasma falls and the patient becomes acidotic. Kussmaul respiration, a deep sighing type of breathing, is seen in all patients with acidosis, usually appearing when the plasma bicarbonate falls below 18 mmol/l. This breathing pattern is due to stimulation of the respiratory centre by the less alkaline plasma and, although it gives the impression of breathlessness, it is not due to lack of oxygen, which is present in normal amounts.

Another important effect of acidosis is interference with normal electrical conduction in the heart, and dysrhythmias may occur. This effect is aggravated by hyperkalaemia, and the combination causes cardiac arrest.

All patients with acute renal failure and most with chronic renal failure, provided it is severe enough, develop acidosis. It is not feasible to prevent ingestion of acid as virtually all diets contain this; also, normal metabolism results in the formation of fixed acid. Acidosis will therefore tend to worsen as time passes. This acidosis can be effectively treated by the administration of sodium bicarbonate, either orally or intravenously as circumstances demand.

Many patients attending chronic renal failure clinics are kept in acid-base equilibrium by taking 1–5 g sodium bicarbonate daily. In acute renal failure dialysis removes excess acid and restores the plasma pH to normal, while in an acutely acidotic patient, who has taken an overdose of aspirin or who is in the diabetic precoma, the intravenous administration of 8.4% sodium bicarbonate solution in calculated amounts will neutralise hydrogen ion, and help avert the danger of dysrhythmias.

4   Protein waste products

These substances are the result of turnover of body tissues and of the utilisation of protein in the diet. They are excreted by the kidneys only and therefore accumulate in all types of renal failure. They fall into three main groups:

(i) *Urea*. This is formed principally from ingested protein. The amount of urea to be disposed of in the urine therefore depends on the amount of protein in the diet. As there is no way of storing protein, any amount greater than the metabolic requirement is changed to urea and excreted. There is always a requirement of about 20 g protein per day, because the daily turnover of tissues is not completely efficient and some is lost; if this loss is not made good from the diet, wasting will occur. The metabolism is always shifted towards catabolism in acutely ill patients, those with fevers and in postoperative patients, resulting in an increase in the rate of protein breakdown. Therefore, these patients form larger amounts of urea per day than they do when their metabolism is in balance. It is inappropriate to starve such patients of dietary protein even though it is known that they cannot fully utilise it, and most of it is broken down to urea. However, if profound wasting is to be avoided protein feeding must continue.

It is possible to devise very low protein diets with an adequate calorie content (Giovanetti type diets) but they are unpalatable and monotonous. The majority of patients default from such diets, which seriously impairs their usefulness. However, these diets do have the advantage of minimising the production of urea, and are sometimes useful in advanced chronic renal failure when dialysis facilities are unobtainable.

When peritoneal dialysis is performed account must always be taken of the losses of protein and amino acids in dialysis fluids. This is always considerable, being at least 0.5–1 g per cycle, and two or three times as much if there is any peritoneal inflammation. In such circumstances, dietary protein may have to be increased to above normal amounts to maintain any semblance of balance and prevent excessive wasting. The limit is usually set by the rather low amounts of protein which most ill patients can tolerate.

When the metabolism shifts back to the anabolic phase on recovery from the acute illness, better utilisation of food protein occurs and the blood urea tends to fall below normal levels.

(ii) *Uric Acid.* This is formed principally from the breaking-down nuclei of rapidly turning over groups of cells. The rate of formation of uric acid is therefore fairly constant unless there is a large change in mitotic activity. Sometimes very large amounts of uric acid are released into the circulation, for example when large numbers of white blood cells are killed simultaneously in the chemotherapeutic treatment of the leukaemias. This can lead to a sudden large rise in the serum uric acid, with deposition of uric acid crystals in the kidneys and elsewhere, occasionally causing acute renal failure.

Acute or chronic renal failure, whatever its cause, leads to high serum uric acid levels because of excretory failure. This is never a problem in acute renal failure, though secondary gout sometimes occurs in chronic renal failure.

(iii) *Creatinine.* This may be considered to be the product of endogenous protein breakdown. In other words it reflects the breakdown of cells in muscle, skin, the uterus, and so on. As this turnover is fairly constant in the normal individual, blood creatinine levels do not fluctuate much. If catabolism increases when renal function is impaired, the creatinine level may rise very rapidly. However creatinine, like urea, is not a toxic substance and does not itself cause symptoms.

When endogenous protein turnover is normal, the state of renal function is indicated by the concentration of creatinine in the serum, which is not affected much by the amount of protein in the diet, unlike blood urea. For example, a patient given a Giovanetti diet may actually reduce his blood urea. This is not due to improved renal function (the Giovanetti diet has no direct effect on the kidneys) but is due to the fact that less unnecessary protein in the food has to be excreted as urea. Measurement of the serum creatinine, which is hardly influenced by the amount of protein in the diet, will then show the true state of affairs.

(iv) *Other protein waste products.* The substances already mentioned (urea, uric acid and creatinine) are important because of the large quantities which accumulate in renal failure. They are not in themselves toxic. However, they are generally used as indicators of the state of the kidneys because they can easily be measured in the hospital laboratory. The symptoms of renal failure are caused by other substances derived from protein breakdown, present in smaller amounts and toxic unless eliminated. They are thought to be the agents which cause such symptoms as vomiting, diarrhoea, anaemia and itching. Most hospital laboratories are not equipped to measure these substances which, however, may safely be assumed to be present when the blood urea or creatinine is found to be raised.

Dialysis

In all patients with acute renal failure the principles of management outlined above will be put into operation, the four groups of functions being considered separately and the appropriate measures taken. In this way the dangerous complications of pulmonary oedema due to overhydration (often misleadingly called 'left ventricular failure'), hyperkalaemia and acidosis will have been avoided. In many patients with postoperative renal failure this conservative management may suffice, as function often recovers on the fourth or fifth day.

If control cannot be maintained in this way, support of renal function with either peritoneal dialysis or with haemodialysis will have to be considered. The choice between the two methods depends on the completeness of the renal shutdown and on the rate of catabolism of the individual patient. Generally, the more severe cases require haemodialysis. These patients have greatly increased catabolism, the blood urea rising by more than 15 mmol (100 mg) per 100 ml per day. Likely candidates are those with much tissue injury due to trauma, burns or sepsis. Patients who have had extensive abdominal surgery, and in whom peritoneal dialysis is not technically feasible, should also be given haemodialysis. It will be found in practice that over half the patients can be managed by peritoneal dialysis.

Haemodialysis

The artificial kidney is fundamentally a filter. It is made from cellulose film ('membrane') which has been rolled to such a thickness that only the smallest molecules can pass through its tiny pores. These include water, electrolytes, acid and all the protein waste products which accumulate in chronic renal failure. Other constituents of the blood, including red and white cells, platelets and plasma proteins, are too large to pass through the membrane. The process is called *dialysis* or ultrafiltration. Some useful plasma constituents such as glucose and amino acids are also small enough to pass through the membrane, but they can readily be replaced in the circulation. When the waste substances have crossed the membrane they dissolve in the dialysing fluid and are carried away to waste.

All artificial kidneys currently in routine use depend on cellulose membranes. Their very different appearances are simply due to different methods of packaging, usually with the object of saving space and improving sterility. The cellulose may be in the form of an envelope, a sausage wound in a spiral, or multiple fine tubes. In all cases, the blood from the patient passes into the space inside the cellulose, which is bathed on the outside by the dialysis fluid. In terms of performance, there is little to choose between different types of artificial kidneys; most acute renal units keep to one or two types with which the staff can become familiar. All types are deliberately inefficient, being designed to effect a gradual reduction in the blood urea over six to eight hours, as too rapid a clearance can result in cerebral oedema with coning and medullary compression, or in cardiac dysrhythmias which can be fatal. This point must be borne in mind if the patient is a child or small adult and the dialysis adjusted to be less efficient. This can be done by slowing the blood flow or, perhaps, by clipping off half of the artificial kidney. However, the frequency of dialysis is not altered to decrease efficiency and in all cases the objective will be to maintain the blood urea below 30 mmol/100 ml (200 mg/100 ml) at all times. Usually this requires daily treatment for about 4–6 hours, depending on the rate of catabolism.

It is usual to obtain the dialysis fluid from a machine which mixes commercially available concentrate with filtered, softened tap water to give an 'ideal' electrolyte solution. The composition is given in Table 4.2. The use of such a solution will return abnormal electrolytes to normal in a single dialysis. The potassium content of dialysing fluid is low or absent because patients with acute renal failure are almost always over-loaded with potassium. If the serum potassium falls after repeated dialysis potassium chloride can be given orally or by injection to correct it.

It is customary to use a dialysate flow of about 500 ml/min, with the popular single-pass artificial kidneys, so 180–200 litres is used per dialysate.

A sufficient flow of blood to obtain a reasonable dialysis is 100–150 ml/min. Flows of this rate can only be conveniently obtained from an artery, either by a temporary indwelling catheter in the femoral artery or, more conveniently, by placement of an arterio-venous shunt in a peripheral artery such as the radial or posterior tibial.

The technique of placement of an arterio-venous shunt is very simple, being only a little more troublesome than an ordinary 'cut-down'. It is best to use tubes with Teflon tips to insert into the blood vessels and these are pushed into flexible silicone rubber catheters which are brought out through the skin. Secure tying of the catheter tips in the vessels is

Table 4.2 The 'ideal' composition of haemodialysis fluid

sodium	136	mmol/l
potassium	1.5	mmol/l
calcium	1.5	mmol/l
chloride	102.3	mmol/l
glucose	11	mmol/l
acetate	40	mmol/l
magnesium	0.8	mmol/l

important, special attention being paid to the vein, which is extremely slippery. The artificial shunt can be used immediately after insertion, when blood is pumped from the arterial catheter with an electric roller-pump. Immediately on leaving the pump, heparin is added to the blood with a syringe pump to prevent clotting in the extracorporeal circulation, and this pump is kept running throughout the dialysis. Usually 15–20 000 i.u. of heparin are required. Some heparin is dialysed out, and some metabolised by the patient. It is desired to keep the patient's clotting time at about 30 minutes (measured in a test tube at the bedside). It is extremely unusual for bleeding problems to arise as a result of giving such doses of heparin in this way, even in traumatised and postsurgical patients, but if necessary a second syringe pump can be used to neutralise the heparin with protamine, just before the blood is returned to the patient.

At the conclusion of the dialysis the arterial and venous ends of the shunt are connected with a plastic connector, and secured with adhesive tape. Arterial blood now flows directly from the artery to the vein, but in such small quantities as not to make any significant difference to the cardiac output. It is not necessary to heparinise the patient to prevent clotting in the shunt, which should be observed hourly for signs of clotting, such as separation of the red blood cells from the plasma in the transparent plastic tube. If this should occur, declotting should be undertaken immediately with a thin plastic cannula attached to a 5 ml syringe, using warm heparinised (1000 u. heparin/l) 0.9 % saline to irrigate the vein and artery. The clot can usually be easily aspirated and flow restored in this way. The vein always gives more trouble than the artery and it may be necessary to force small residual clots into the vein in order to clear it. This seems to cause no trouble and presumably the clot is absorbed. However, it is dangerous to force clots into arteries especially in the arm as the capacity of the forearm arteries is only about 10 ml and a clot can be forced from the arm to the brain causing sudden death. If the artery seems irretrievably blocked, another arterial catheter should be inserted.

It is possible to remove water overload from a patient with an artificial kidney by adjusting the pressure on each side of the membrane, and 5–6 litres can be removed from an overhydrated patient in this way in each dialysis, provided the blood pressure remains stable. It is thus highly effective as a means of treating pulmonary oedema.

Other water-soluble substances in the blood behave like urea, provided their molecular size is sufficiently small. Potassium is easily and rapidly extracted and water-soluble drugs such as phenobarbitone and aspirin are rapidly washed out. Many other drugs, such as digoxin, are not affected because they are bound to protein molecules which cannot pass the membrane. Others, such as many of the antidepressants, are dissolved in body fat and are not available for dialysis. The use of the artificial kidney in clearing the plasma of poisons and of overdoses of drugs is therefore limited.

It must be stressed that haemodialysis is not safely undertaken by those without training in the technique. The mortality in experienced and well-equipped haemodialysis units approaches 50 % in all cases of acute renal failure and this figure is undoubtedly exceeded by those less experienced. Patients requiring haemodialysis should be transferred to a special unit.

Peritoneal dialysis

The technique of peritoneal dialysis is simple. Under local anaesthesia, a plastic cannula is introduced into the peritoneal cavity by use of a trocar. The most suitable positions are shown in Fig. 4.1. About 10 ml of 2 % lignocaine is used, first raising a weal in the skin then infiltrating the subcutaneous tissues as the needle is advanced vertically towards the peritoneum. On reaching the peritoneum the patient feels a pricking sensation, and the needle is withdrawn slightly so that the area can be thoroughly infiltrated. An incision 0.6 cm long is made through the skin weal with a scalpel blade; it must pass through the full thickness of the skin. Healing is rapid if the incision has been made in the direction of the skin folds.

The trocar is placed in the cannula and introduced vertically with a to-and-fro screwing motion. As long as muscle is avoided, advancement is easy until the peritoneum is reached, when resistance is often met. The

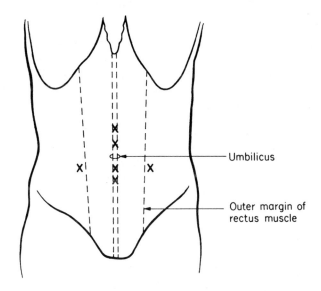

X suitable positions for insertion of peritoneal dialysis catheter

Fig. 4.1 The usual sites of insertion of a peritoneal dialysis catheter

consistency of the peritoneum resembles that of thick wet cardboard, and it may be necessary to continue the screwing motion for a minute or two before the very definite sensation of the peritoneum giving way is felt. When this occurs, pressure is immediately relaxed and the trocar is not advanced any further. The cannula is now advanced into the peritoneal cavity, preferably towards the pelvis. The patient can often feel the position of the cannula tip and say where it is. Sometimes discomfort is caused if the cannula tip is adjacent to the rectum, but it should not be moved by the operator as the discomfort is temporary and the cannula moves about anyway under the influence of peristalsis.

When almost the whole length of the cannula has been inserted, the protruding end is fixed with tapes so that it cannot slip completely into the peritonium. There is no need to insert a purse-string suture. The peritoneal fluid reservoir is now connected and the fluid allowed to run freely, having been warmed previously to body temperature. It should run in a continuous stream if the cannula has been correctly placed. Cycles of two litres are run as rapidly as possible to obtain the best results, the return from the peritoneal cavity being by siphonage into a closed drainage system (Fig. 4.2).

Sometimes it is found at the beginning of a peritoneal dialysis that not all the fluid returns. This is usually due to the fluid having tracked into the

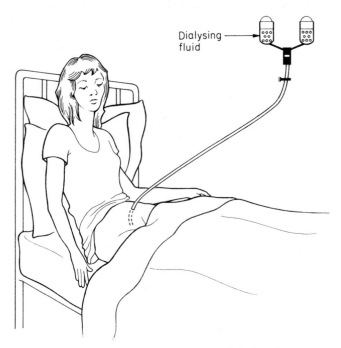

Dialysing fluid

Fig. 4.2 Positioning of a peritoneal dialysis catheter

pelvis, the intestines then floating up to obstruct the cannula. It is usually best to ignore this fluid for the first three cycles. After this amount has been given a channel will form and the return volumes will then exceed the amounts of dialysate administered so that balance is achieved after a few more cycles. The amounts administered and returned should be accurately charted, and a deficit of four litres or more in the return should prompt alteration in the position of the patient with the object of bringing the fluid into contact with the cannula. If this fails to achieve the desired results, the external tubes should be examined for fibrin blockage. This can sometimes be removed by syringing and its further formation prevented by adding 100–200 units of heparin to each dialysis cycle.

If the cannula has accidentally been placed subcutaneously, the peritoneum not being penetrated, oedema of the body wall will occur when the dialysing fluid is run in. A new cannula should be inserted at another site. Occasionally the large bowel is perforated by the cannula and profuse watery diarrhoea occurs when the dialysing fluid is run in. In this case the cannula should be withdrawn and a fresh one inserted elsewhere, the dialysis being continued. If the returns become cloudy an antibiotic such as ampicillin can be added to the dialysate. Neomycin must not be used intraperitoneally as it may cause respiratory arrest. It is not necessary to perform a laparotomy because the site of perforation seals itself as soon as the cannula is withdrawn. Occasionally a pericolic abscess develops but more usually there are no sequelae to this accident, provided that dialysis (and peritoneal lavage) are continued.

Peritoneal dialysis should not be performed on unconscious or drowsy patients until the stomach is emptied or an airway secured, preferably with an endotracheal tube, because of the risk of vomiting and inhalation in such patients. Recent abdominal surgery is not necessarily a contra-indication, though this will depend upon the nature of the operation performed. Leakage may occur through surgical wounds and drain holes but does not harm, apart from wetting the bed clothes. This nuisance can be alleviated by the use of ileostomy bags.

Continued peritoneal dialysis is sometimes associated with peritonitis after three or four days. The return fluid then looks milky or hazy with purulence. A specimen is sent for culture (usually *Escherichia coli* is grown) and an antibiotic such as ampicillin 100 mg is added to each dialysis cycle, which continues without interruption. When the return has become clear, and remained so for several cycles, the antibiotic is discontinued. It is not necessary to give parenteral antibiotics.

It is not usually possible to reduce the blood urea below 25 mmol/100 ml (150 mg/100 ml) by peritoneal dialysis, and about 30 mmol/100 ml (200 mg/100 ml) is a suitable target. When this level is reached dialysis is discontinued, leaving the catheter in place until it is required again. It is often possible to maintain the urea at satisfactory levels by dialysing during the day only (e.g. 20 cycles) leaving the nights undisturbed.

Avoidance of acute renal failure

Although some cases of acute renal failure have recognisable single causes (such as prolonged hypotension) most patients have suffered at least one other additional causal factor, which is usually recognisable from their history. The clinical situation is usually divisible into predisposing factors and precipitating factors. Some of these are given in Table 4.3. It is apparent that when the risk of a particular situation is appreciated, avoiding action can sometimes be taken. For example, it is unwise to operate on a jaundiced patient who has been vomiting without first rehydrating the patient and restoring the electrolytes to normal before inducing the anaesthetic. Similarly, in established cases of acute renal failure, factors already mentioned should be sought and corrected first as far as is possible. In this connection the duration of the metabolic insult may be critical. It is pertinent to mention the experience of the American medical services in the Vietnam war, who showed that prompt restoration of blood volume in a battle casualty could avert the development of tubular necrosis if carried out within five hours of the wounding. The nature of the transfusion is less important and although blood is best in that particular situation plasma, plasma substitutes (such as high molecular weight dextran) or even saline is better than nothing. If resuscitation was delayed beyond five hours acute renal failure was about ten times more common.

In addition to the factors mentioned above, when renal failure develops postoperatively there is always a strong suspicion that a surgical complication may be contributing. Leakage from surgical anastomosis is a common cause; internal haemorrhage with shock is another. In such cases, the patient seldom survives without further surgical intervention. Even if corrective surgery is done, the mortality rate is still over 50 %. The diagnosis of the nature of the surgical complication is often extremely

---

Table 4.3   Factors which may lead to acute renal failure

Predisposing factors:
   pregnancy
   jaundice, especially obstructive
   any chronic renal disease
   sodium deficiency
   dehydration
   fixed hypertension
   poor cardiac output
Precipitating factors:
   blood loss
   gram negative bacteraemia
   disseminated intravascular coagulation
   chemical toxins (carbon tetrachloride etc.)
   nephrotoxic antibiotics

difficult or impossible before laparotomy. A second operation will often aggravate the renal failure, making a partial tubular necrosis complete, but this consideration should not be allowed to influence surgical decision-making as acute renal failure should always be regarded as a treatable and recoverable condition.

Course of acute renal failure

Once control of the immediate situation has been gained and the first dialysis sessions have normalised the patient's biochemistry and fluid status, the management falls naturally into two parts. Initially, the management of associated lesions will continue by consultation with the relevant specialists in anaesthetics, general and orthopaedic surgery, obstetrics and all other interested parties. Usually considerations of dialysis will take precedence until secretion of urine begins, but it is certainly possible in most patients to carry out most other therapeutic procedures during the period of tubular necrosis.

So far as the renal failure is concerned, the patient is considered to be anephric. The fluid intake is therefore strictly controlled to prevent over hydration and the amounts of sodium and potassium given must be strictly limited. The blood urea is controlled by dialysis, usually performed daily or on alternate days. In most cases, the period of anuria lasts about 21 days, though occasionally up to six weeks can elapse before secretion of urine recommences. The initial urine is dilute but copious, and a diuresis of up to three or four litres a day is often seen. There is often a considerable loss of potassium and sodium in this diuretic phase, necessitating replacement orally or intravenously. After about a week, the concentrating ability begins to return and is slowly restored to normal over the next few weeks.

If a diuresis does not begin within three or four weeks, doubts about the viability of the kidneys may be entertained. These can be resolved only by time or by renal biopsy, which will indicate whether recovery can occur. It can then be decided whether it is appropriate to continue dialysis treatment or whether transfer to a chronic dialysis centre should be arranged.

5

Metabolic Disorders

Liver failure

The metabolic and excretory functions of the liver are so numerous that it is not at present possible to substitute them all by artificial means. The care of patients suffering from liver failure is aimed at maintaining essential functions until recovery occurs spontaneously. A good functional recovery can occur even when most of the liver cells have been completely destroyed because of the capacity of those cells which remain to regenerate useful functioning tissue. Although the liver may be anatomically abnormal and liable to further damage by distortion from continuing fibrosis, a regenerated liver can sustain a normal life.

The liver receives two blood supplies. The first is the portal supply which delivers all the blood draining the gastro-intestinal tract and which contains all classes of absorbed food substances. Most of these need modification by liver cells, while others pass through the liver into the systemic circulation. Many bacteria and their metabolic products also reach the liver from the large bowel by the portal vein; these are filtered from the blood and destroyed or detoxified by the liver cells. For this purpose the major portion of the reticulo-endothelial system is located in the liver. Finally, ingested foreign substances such as drugs arrive at the liver in the portal blood and may be metabolised and excreted by the liver, or pass through it unchanged.

A second blood supply arrives at the liver by the hepatic artery, supplying the oxygen necessary for metabolism. Parenterally administered drugs arrive by this route, possibly for conjugation and excretion by either the liver or by the kidneys, sometimes by both.

Although the hepatic artery is small, the liver, which it supplies, is very sensitive to reduction in arterial blood flow. Obviously ligation of the hepatic artery causes hepatic necrosis, but any fall in hepatic artery perfusion, caused by reduced cardiac output, is likely to cause damage to or even necrosis of the centrilobular liver cells. Liver transaminases released from the damaged cells are readily detected in the plasma. If the liver function has already been put at risk, for example by cirrhosis, a lowered cardiac output can precipitate liver failure in this way. Maintenance of the cardiac output is therefore an important part of the management of the patient with hepatic failure.

In addition to the detoxifying, conjugating and excretory functions, numerous metabolic functions occur principally in the liver: it is the only site of formation of both albumin and urea, so the blood concentrations of these substances can be seriously reduced in liver failure; it contains the supply of glycogen which can be broken down to maintain blood sugar concentrations; it metabolises hormones; it produces and excretes into the intestine bile salts and bile acids which are essential for the absorption of fat and of the fat-soluble vitamins A, D, E and K; it plays an essential role in the regulation of serum cholesterol; and it manufactures fibrinogen and other coagulation factors.

Liver failure can be either acute or chronic. Chronic liver failure is often punctuated by episodes of acute failure requiring hospital admission. As is the case in chronic renal failure, not all liver functions are lost equally simultaneously. Instead, there is great variation in the clinical picture depending upon which functions are mostly impaired in a particular patient. These episodes are commonly precipitated by blood loss, usually from gastro-intestinal bleeding, or by intercurrent infection, or by trauma, either surgical or accidental. In acute hepatic failure a major proportion of all functions is lost simultaneously and completely, so that the patient's life is at risk. Precipitating factors include infective hepatitis, the ingestion of toxic substances (particularly paracetamol) and surgery of the biliary tract, especially in the presence of bacterial infection. Additionally, it must always be borne in mind that chronic liver disease can present for the first time as acute hepatic failure.

Management of acute hepatic failure

The objective of management is to support life until recovery of the liver occurs spontaneously. Regeneration of hepatocytes can begin within two weeks of the onset of acute hepatic failure. It is not usually possible to tell at the outset which patients will be able to regenerate their liver cells, and liver biopsy is of no help in this respect. It is simplest to separate the management into the areas in which the patient is monitored:

(i) **Encephalopathy**. This is usually the most important symptom, as its outcome determines the patient's fate. Clinical estimates are made of the state of consciousness and charted four-hourly. The stages shown in Table 5.1 are generally used. The importance of staging the level of consciousness lies in its prognostic value, as the recovery rate diminishes with increasing encephalopathy and less than 10% of those patients entering stage 4 make a recovery.

Table 5.1 Stages of encephalopathy

Stage	
1	Confused, inappropriate mood
2	Drowsy, disorientated, possibly manic
3	Stupor, rousable
4	Unrousable, may respond to painful stimuli

Several factors are important in the production of hepatic encephalopathy:

(a) *Intoxication with ammonia* and with other substances derived from bacterial metabolism in the colon. In the normal individual, bacterial products from the large intestine are extracted from the portal blood as it passes through the liver. Of particular importance is ammonia, which is produced by the action of bacteria on protein in the colon and which normally never reaches the systemic circulation. However, in liver damage the blood ammonia level rises and is associated with impairment of consciousness. The degree of impairment roughly correlates with the concentration of blood ammonia.

Other substances, originating in the gut, gain access to the circulation in liver failure and affect the level of consciousness. These include 'false neurotransmitter' substances derived from protein metabolism which have pharmacological actions on the brain and are responsible for symptoms such as confusion, ataxia and tremor. Amino acids whose blood concentrations are normally controlled by liver cells are found in increased concentration and certain of these, especially methionine, appear to be associated with worsening encephalopathy. For this reason the intravenous amino acid mixtures available at present are contra-indicated in acute hepatic failure.

Liver failure patients should have their colons washed out by enemas to remove the material from which ammonia is formed. In addition, the non-absorbable carbohydrate lactulose can be given as a syrup in amounts deliberately sufficient to cause mild diarrhoea. Usually this can be achieved with 100–150 g daily in divided doses. This produces an acid stool which traps any ammonia formed in the bowel so that it is passed per rectum, and does not gain access to the circulation.

It is customary to give neomycin syrup 1 g six-hourly orally so as to reduce the colonic bacterial population and thereby reduce the amount of bacterial toxins formed. This treatment introduces a risk, albeit remote, of superinfection of the bowel with resistant organisms. Furthermore, although neomycin is commonly regarded as a non-absorbable antibiotic variable amounts are in fact absorbed from the intestine, especially if it is inflamed or otherwise abnormal. As the drug is profoundly nephrotoxic, its use should not continue beyond 48 hours.

Tetracycline related antibiotics should not be used for bowel sterilisation purposes as they are absorbed, nephrotoxic and under intense suspicion as rare causative agents of acute hepatic failure.

For the duration of the hepatic encephalopathy, protein should be eliminated from the diet, and protein balance should be maintained by infusion of blood and blood products.

(b) *Sedative drugs.* If possible these substances should be avoided in acute hepatic encephalopathy. Such patients are often extremely sensitive to sedation, even in small doses. These drugs are often the cause of the encephalopathy in the first place, and regularly depress the conscious level by one or two stages. Indeed they are usually used to convert a stage 1 or 2 hyperactive patient to stage 3. This is a therapeutic disaster. It cannot be too strongly emphasised that the primary object of treatment of hepatic encephalopathy is the maintenance and improvement of the conscious level.

(ii) **Bleeding and coagulation.** As the liver plays a central role in the production of fibrinogen and of clotting factors, disorders of the clotting mechanism are very common in hepatic failure and are second in importance to encephalopathy in determining the outcome. Intravascular coagulation is usually present at least within the vessels of the liver and may be disseminated throughout the circulation. It is thought to be due to contact of the blood with necrotic liver cells. The consumption of clotting factors by this mechanism can lead to hypofibrinogenaemia, and this may cause generalised bleeding. This is particularly noticeable in the skin and mucous membranes, with a generalised capillary ooze into the intestine. The loss of blood further impairs the circulation, increasing hypoxic damage, while the blood in the intestine acts as a protein meal which thus still further exacerbates the encephalopathy.

This situation should be anticipated as far as possible by seeking laboratory evidence of intravascular coagulation on admission and at least daily afterwards. If such evidence is found, intravenous heparin infusion is begun, under laboratory control, to prevent further clotting. At the same time an infusion of fresh frozen plasma is begun to provide fibrinogen and those clotting factors which the damaged liver cells can no longer synthesise in sufficient quantity (Chapter 8).

Bleeding due to lack of clotting factors and coagulation failure often takes the form of capillary oozing in many different sites, especially the skin and the gastro-intestinal mucous membranes. It is almost impossible to estimate the quantity of such blood loss and a patient may suffer volume depletion and impairment of cardiac output from this cause. Therefore, it is essential in such patients to use the central venous pressure as a guide to blood replacement. Patients with hepatic encephalopathy are particularly vulnerable to a low cardiac output.

As the cause of the bleeding state is invariably complex, and involves platelet consumption and lack of clotting factor formation by sick hepatocytes, fresh frozen plasma is the best transfusion in these circumstances. The blood volume and haemoglobin should be maintained at normal levels and daily estimates made of fibrinogen degradation products, fibrinogen titres, platelets and haemoglobin levels.

(iii) **Hypoglycaemia.** The liver is the principal source of the blood glucose. In acute hepatic failure profound hypoglycaemia may occur as a result of the liver's failure to make sufficient glucose from glycogen, and it may appear with remarkable suddenness. Obviously hypoglycaemia causes coma in its own right; it also exacerbates hepatic encephalopathy. Hypoglycaemia can be prevented with an infusion of dextrose and this is usually indicated anyway as a means of providing calories. If for any reason a non-dextrose infusion is employed, the blood glucose must be estimated and charted hourly, and any fall below 4.4 mmol/l (80 mg/dl) treated by dextrose infusion. It is convenient to monitor the blood glucose by means of 'Dextrostix' at the bedside. Many ICUs continue this estimation as a routine in liver failure whether a dextrose drip is given or not.

(iv) **Acidosis.** A metabolic acidosis is often seen in liver failure; it is usually due to the accumulation of lactic acid. Its presence can be confirmed by the measurement of serum lactate but unfortunately many laboratories do not offer this service. In such cases the presence of a lactic acidosis can be strongly suspected from the serum electrolyte results by calculation of the 'anion gap' from the serum electrolytes (page 34). This relies on the fact that $[Na^+ + K^+] - [Cl^- + HCO_3^-]$ is less than 20 mmol/l in the normal individual; if it is greater than 20, the difference is assumed to be due to lactic acid accumulation, although other causes (e.g. sodium carbenicillin and severe dehydration) should be considered. Correction is made with intravenous sodium bicarbonate.

(v) **Renal failure.** A degree of renal failure often accompanies liver failure; the onset of anuria is an extremely ominous sign and usually heralds death. The presence of renal failure is sometimes partly obscured by the fact that urea is made by the liver exclusively, and a failed liver may not be able to perform this task. The blood urea then shows very little increase even though the kidneys are not functioning. It may be necessary to support the kidneys by peritoneal dialysis. Curiously, dialysis does not assist in the management of hepatic failure, even though many of the clinical features are thought to be due to the presence of dialysable toxic substances such as ammonia and amino acids.

(vi) **Respiratory failure.** Essentially caused by cerebral depression, respiratory failure worsens the prognosis. It is diagnosed by blood gas estimation, and its treatment is on standard lines (page 76). Patients with liver failure whose treatment requires artificial ventilation do not often recover.

(vii) **Drugs and hepatic failure.** As the management of hepatic failure is expectant no particular drugs are indicated. Corticosteroids do not influence the development of the disease and do not improve liver function in any measurable way. As they encourage opportunistic infection and may cause gastrointestinal haemorrhage, they are contra-indicated. No antibiotics, except neomycin, are indicated unless sepsis occurs. Even the place of neomycin is not secure; it is predictably absorbed from the gut and has been known to cause renal tubular necrosis when given orally. However, this risk is small, and the benefits probably outweigh the disadvantages of the drug. It should be discontinued as soon as possible to prevent super-infection with opportunistic organisms.

It is customary to give vitamin supplements in hepatic failure, especially vitamin K, and these can do no harm.

Diabetes

In diabetic pre-coma and coma two metabolic abnormalities occur. In the first place, failure of glucose utilisation leads to increasing levels in the blood. This high blood glucose acts as an osmotic diuretic and large volumes of dilute urine are passed. The urine contains quantities of sodium and, especially, potassium. The patient, feeling thirsty, drinks increased amounts of fluids which do not usually contain much sodium or potassium. Thus, while water balance is maintained, sodium and potassium concentrations in the patient's blood begin to fall. The process may continue for several days, the serum sodium being made up from the extracellular fluids and the potassium from the intracellular stores. The sodium loss causes hypotension and nausea; the potassium loss causes profound weakness. Eventually the patient may be too weak and nauseated to replace the water loss but the diuresis continues under the influence of the high blood sugar and a clinical picture of dehydration and electrolyte loss results.

At the same time, in the absence of sufficient insulin, fat is catabolised as an energy source in the place of carbohydrate. Under these conditions the fat catabolism is incomplete, and results in the formation of ketone bodies, one of which (acetone) can be smelled on the patient's breath. Also found are aceto-acetic acid and β-hydroxybuturic acid. These substances, accumulating in the plasma, cause a metabolic acidosis which in turn interferes with metabolism throughout the organism causing the typical acidotic respiration and eventually impairment of consciousness. Ketone bodies are water soluble and may be detected in the urine by simple tests.

Treatment is directed at replacing lost fluid and electrolyte, correcting the acidosis and giving sufficient insulin to convert catabolism back to the utilisation of glucose in place of fat. The keto acids are not attacked directly; they can be left to be filtered into the urine or metabolised in the usual way in the presence of insulin.

The most important immediate treatment is the replacement of fluid and electrolyte. This is done by the rapid infusion of normal saline to which potassium chloride has been added, at about the rate of 15 mmol/l depending on the serum potassium. There is always a large potassium deficit in diabetic pre-coma and it may be necessary to give extra potassium chloride, particularly as potassium rapidly withdraws into cells once insulin treatment has begun. Potassium in amounts of 15–75 mmol/h may be necessary, and treatment must be controlled by frequent laboratory estimations which are the only reliable guide. It is not safe to rely on the electrocardiogram to give evidence of hypokalaemia as it is usually a late sign and sometimes does not even appear.

The state of hydration may be reliably monitored by means of a CVP line; however, as the patient's conscious level usually recovers during adequate treatment and as there is little danger of causing fluid overload in the presence of normal renal function, a CVP line may not always be necessary.

It is best to give insulin as monocomponent insulin by continuous intravenous infusion. Insulins other than soluble insulin must not be given in this way. The insulin is given by infusion pump at the rate of four units of insulin per hour. This is a very low dose compared with the amounts given in the traditional four-hourly routines, the reason being that in the older method about 90 % of the insulin was never used but was broken down by the liver. Furthermore, the amounts of insulin given by the 'sliding scale' subcutaneous or intramuscular insulin technique were often large and sometimes produced hypoglycaemia in a highly un-predictable way, depending on uncertain rates of absorption. With the continuous infusion method small changes with smoother management is obtained throughout a critical period.

If the patient has become very dehydrated before treatment has begun, the circulating blood volume will be low and tissue anoxia is sometimes present. Lactic acidosis will then contribute to overall acidosis. It can be diagnosed by measuring the serum lactate, or its presence can be inferred by estimating the 'anion gap' (page 34). The presence of lactic acidosis is an indication for adding a calculated amount of sodium bicarbonate to the intravenous infusion. Lactic acidosis is particularly likely to be a feature if phenformin has been used for the diabetic management of the patient before the coma began.

As well as treatment of the diabetic coma, the precipitating cause will have to be identified and treated. Usually this is simply a neglect to take the prescribed amount of insulin, but sometimes intercurrent infections such a pneumonia or pyelonephritis cause a stable diabetic to become unstable. In this connection it may be mentioned that diabetics are more susceptible to intercurrent infection than most other patients. This is not an indication for 'prophylactic' antibiotics, but it should certainly make one think twice about routine bladder catheterisation simply for the convenience of fluid balance charts. The renal tract, particularly the kidneys of diabetics, is peculiarly susceptible to ascending infection, which may cause serious or even fatal damage ranging from un-controllable pyelonephritis to papillary necrosis. Catheterisation should, therefore, be avoided if management is possible without it.

Hyperosmolar diabetic coma

This unusual variant of diabetic coma occurs in those who have drunk quantities of sweetened fluids during the period of dehydration.

Lemonade sweetened with glucose is frequently the beverage employed. The blood glucose rises to very high levels (normal serum concentrations are 3.3–7.0 mmol/l) and the rise in keto acids is small or absent. The high glucose level of the blood raises its osmolarity and this causes it to extract water from the extracellular space. The extra water is promptly excreted by the kidneys. Thus, the concentration, or osmolarity of the serum keeps increasing from the normal 275–300 mOsmol/l to perhaps 400–425 mOsmol/l. When this stage has been reached about 7 litres of water and about 500 mmol of sodium has been lost. As 7 litres of physiological (0.9%) saline contain 1050 mmol of sodium, 0.45% saline must be employed for fluid replacement. If 0.9% saline is used the additional sodium may raise the osmolarity to a level at which the brain is permanently damaged. The essential point is that more water than solute must be given to dilute the hyperosmolar serum.

Hypoglycaemic coma

This is caused by an overdose of insulin or of an oral hypoglycaemic agent such as phenformin. As glucose is essential for brain function, prolonged hypoglycaemia may cause irreversible brain damage. The situation is controlled, usually dramatically, by giving intravenous glucose. Water and electrolyte imbalance are not a feature of hypoglycaemic coma.

Hypoglycaemia may also contribute to the impaired consciousness of hepatic coma because of the lack of new glucose formation by the damaged liver. It is essential to check the blood sugar frequently when acute liver damage is suspected in intensive care patients.

Addison's disease

In this condition, which has now become rare, the secretion of corticosteriods by the adrenal glands is deficient. The principal effect of this deficiency is on the kidney, which cannot retain salt in the absence of corticosteroids and hence excessive amounts are lost in the urine; these losses of salt exceed the amount ingested by the patient. The serum sodium and chloride concentrations fall to low values (about 110 mmol/l of sodium and 60 mmol/l of chloride) and the blood volume is reduced. This in turn leads to a low blood pressure which is often below 100 mmHg (13.3 kPa) systolic. The patient is weak and wasted, anorexia and vomiting maybe occuring due to the low sodium; at the same time, sodium continues to appear in the urine. The situation of sodium appearing in the urine when the serum sodium is low is highly characteristic of Addison's disease, provided the kidneys are normal.

In this low sodium state the patient is vulnerable to any condition which causes even minor volume depletion. Vomiting and diarrhoea are frequently the precipitating factors of shock (Addisonian crisis) because of the fluid and electrolyte loss that they cause. If adequate substitution is not given the patient may die.

All the major physiological defects in Addison's disease can be reversed by giving salt in sufficient quantity to overtake the urinary leak. In the case of Addisonian crisis saline is given intravenously to correct the shock. Corticosteroid therapy alone is not useful as it does not replace the lost salt, though it will certainly prevent further leakage from the kidney. Indeed, it is not necessary to give corticosteroids at all as it is easy to infuse saline at a greater rate than the kidneys can lose it. Care must be taken not to over-transfuse, as the cardiac output is low and the heart is small in Addison's disease, so it is easy to precipitate pulmonary oedema.

It is convenient to continue therapy with corticosteroids alone, using them for their salt-retaining effect. An oral dose of 25 mg cortisone acetate daily is usually sufficient. During intercurrent infection it is customary to increase the dose; more importantly, at these times the salt intake should be increased.

The treatment of Addisonian crisis illustrates the very limited role that corticosteroids play in the treatment of volume-depletion shock, where they can be dispensed with completely provided sufficient salt is administered. It is salutary to remember that the present vogue for administering ever-increasing doses of corticosteroids to shocked patients had its origin in the treatment of Addison's disease. It cannot be too strongly emphasised that the treatment of volume depletion is restoration of the blood volume with fluid and electrolytes, and corticosteroids make almost no contribution in this respect. Furthermore, their encouragement of peptic ulceration and opportunistic infection usually contra-indicates their use. The widespread practice of giving up to 1 g of methyl prednisolone to shocked patients, sometimes even before setting up an intravenous infusion, is deplorable.

The condition of *salt-losing nephritis* is in all respects similar to Addison's disease, except that the kidneys are unable to respond to corticosteroids because they are already diseased. Sufficient salt must be given orally or infusion to overtake the leak; this treatment then becomes a permanent feature of the patient's life.

Thyrotoxic crisis

In this very rare condition, extreme overactivity of the thyroid gland gives rise to the syndrome of thyrotoxic crisis or 'storm'. The clinical features are those of sympathetic nervous system overactivity, with marked tachycardia, sweating, flushing and sometimes hyperpyrexia. There may be heart failure due to the extreme rapidity of the ventricular rate; the cardiac output of most adults begins to fall when the rate exceeds about

160 beats/min even if the ventricles are normal because insufficient time remains for ventricular filling. Rates of around 200 beats/min are seen in thyrotoxic cases.

Treatment consists of reducing sympathetic overactivity with adrenergic blocking agents such as propranolol. This controls the dangerous circulatory abnormalities, slowing the heart rate so that the output can increase and reversing the extreme vasodilatation. Cooling may be necessary if the temperature is over 40°C. Circulatory support with intravenous infusions may also be necessary. The patient is extremely restless and anxious, and sedation with phenothiazine or benzodiazepine drugs is given. Corticosteroids are not indicated and aspirin, which has sometimes been used as an antipyretic in this condition, is definitely contra-indicated as it, too, uncouples oxidative phosphorylation, and may exacerbate the clinical state.

Treatment to prevent the formation of further thyroid hormone should begin as soon as possible. This is done by putting sodium iodide 1–2 g 6-hourly into the intravenous infusion. When the patient is fit enough, antithyroid oral treatment with carbimazole 15 mg 8-hourly should be started.

Thyroid crises are often precipitated by intercurrent infection and evidence of this should be sought so that treatment for it can be started.

Myxoedema coma

This complication of thyroid underactivity may complicate very long-standing cases and is due to the almost complete absence of thyroid secretion. The patient is usually elderly and there is a history of progressive inactivity. Often there has been a precipitating factor such as intercurrent infection or myocardial infarction. Cold injury is frequently a precipitating factor, and is also a result of myxoedema. The cardiac output is low with bradycardia, which can be mistaken clinically for heart block. Hypothermia is common. The respiratory rate is often slow. The usual clinical features of myxoedema are present and are often in a grossly exaggerated form. In particular, there is often a pericardial effusion though without tamponade. Coronary artery disease is very common indeed. Hypoglycaemia is frequent.

Treatment consists of supportive therapy and tri-iodothyronine 10 μg daily. This is usually given orally as it may precipitate a fatal dysrhythmia if given intravenously. Warming, if necessary, should be done slowly by means of blankets not by the application of external heat. The dose of tri-iodothyronine is increased slowly as the patient improves. When the metabolic rate increases previously hidden disabilities (such as coronary artery disease producing severe angina) may begin to appear, and sometimes prove fatal. It may be necessary to give corticosteroids if the origin of the myxoedema is a pituitary lesion, when it can be assumed (or better still proved by measurement of the serum cortisol concentration) that the adrenals are relatively inactive. Otherwise, corticosteroids are not indicated.

Pancreatitis

This devastating condition is due to acute inflammation of the pancreas with activation of its digestive enzymes, which are released into the circulation. It causes severe upper abdominal and upper back pain, often made worse by lying flat. There is usually a great deal of vomiting, sometimes sufficient to cause electrolyte depletion. Frequently there is associated disease of the liver and bile ducts, especially obstructive gallstones. Sometimes there is no preceding history and the condition affects previously healthy people.

The release of activated pancreatic enzymes into the tissues causes local tissue digestion and massive interstitial blood and fluid loss into the retroperitoneal space. This sometimes amounts to eight or ten litres, mostly derived from the circulating blood volume. In addition, enzymes are released into the circulation where they cause widespread damage. Particularly noticeable is lipase, which attacks fat causing fat necrosis. This is sometimes palpable as nodules in fatty subcutaneous tissue, especially in the neck. The digested fat absorbs calcium from the blood and may cause hypocalcaemia with tetany.

Release of trypsin into the circulation causes widespread tissue damage due to protein digestion. This contributes to the general toxaemia. Amylase is also released and is readily detected in the blood.

The combination of these enzymes, the hypovolaemia and the presence of the products of protein breakdown in the circulation sometimes causes acute renal failure.

There is no effective treatment for pancreatitis and the objective is therefore to provide support until recovery occurs. The blood volume is restored with blood and plasma, using a CVP line for guidance. Often very large amounts are required, the transfused fluid leaking through damaged capillaries and into retroperitoneal space. Peritoneal dialysis may be useful as it removes free enzymes and greatly aids the attainment of electrolyte balance. It is probably preferable to haemodialysis even when acute renal failure is present as haemodialysis does not remove useful amounts of enzyme.

Relapse is common in acute pancreatitis and the prognosis on present lines of treatment is poor.

6

Poisoning

Although more than 100 000 patients are admitted to hospital each year in England and Wales with a diagnosis of poisoning, only a small proportion is seriously ill. The majority can be adequately cared for and survive in a general medical ward, relatively few requiring the resources of an Intensive Care Unit.

Moreover, truly accidental poisoning is rare and generally occurs in children under the age of about five, who can be especially in danger if they ingest an overdose of tablets or capsules left within their indiscriminating reach. Again, only a small number needs intensive care. The major incidence of poisoning occurs in adults who deliberately indulge in swallowing an excess of medicines, commonly in tablet or capsule form. Some are determinedly suicidal and most of them are successful. Those who are not usually qualify for intensive management. Most adults taking overdoses, however, are not resolved on self-destruction and are referred to as para-suicidal. Usually they swallow a modest quantity of whatever medicine they choose, though a few are careless about dosage and render themselves seriously ill.

The primary objective of intensive care of the poisoned patient is to maintain life by support of the circulatory and respiratory systems. The secondary objective is to minimise the effect of the poisonous substance by accelerating its removal from the body. In a few cases, when the identity of the poison is accurately known, a specific antidote can be administered. Knowledge of the identity and quantity of the poison is therefore useful and as much information as possible should be collected by questioning relatives, friends and other possible witnesses. Frequently it is found that a mixture of drugs has been taken, some of unknown identity, and very often only the approximate quantity is known. In serious attempts at suicide the information offered by the patient is often unreliable, whereas in the more common dramatic gesture without serious intent the patient will often volunteer precise information.

Aetiology

Because of their motives, these self-poisoners characteristically select psychotropic drugs for their purposes—hypnotics, sedatives, tranquillisers, antidepressants and analgesics, nearly all of which have the property of rendering the patient unconscious and depressing respiration. It is not essential, as a routine, to identify accurately the poison involved since the circumstantial evidence for poisoning is usually adequate.

Examination of specimens of urine, blood and stomach contents by the emergency analytical laboratory should be resorted to only when management might be modified if the agent were precisely recognised, or where a case of coma is undiagnosed but poisoning is suspected.

The symptoms and signs of most drugs taken in overdose are a reflection of their actions in normal dosage. A few drugs in overdose produce characteristic patterns which may help in the diagnosis. For example, barbiturates and phenothiazines can cause respiratory depression, hypotension and hypothermia. Skin blisters occur in patients who have ingested barbiturates, glutethimide, methaqualone, tricyclic antidepressants and meprobamate or have inhaled carbon monoxide. The blisters are characteristically found in sites where pressure has been exerted between two skin surfaces, such as interdigital clefts and inner aspects of knees. Narcotic drugs produce the characteristic pin-point pupils, which should dilate with the administration of the specific opiate-antagonist naloxone.

The development of cardiac dysrhythmias may suggest that the patient has ingested a tricyclic antidepressant compound. These drugs also have anti-cholinergic properties, thus there may be a dry mouth, dilated pupils and a dry feel to the skin.

An overdose of aspirin produces a common pattern; the patient may be admitted with rapid 'acidotic' breathing, excessive sweating and he may complain of tinnitus.

The mouth should be inspected in a poisoned patient as there may be evidence of corrosive burns to the mucosa. This will be found with strong acids, alkalis and with paraquat.

Many common poisons produce no special identifying features. For these patients it is more important to assess the severity of the poisoning. Recordings of the minute and tidal volumes are very important.

Paracetamol poisoning produces no characteristic picture in the early stages. It is important that this poison is recognised early since safe and effective antidotes are available, preventing the late sequelae of severe liver damage. Most emergency departments have kits for the estimation of serum paracetamol.

Management

The principles for managing any case of poisoning are based on conservative support and the preservation of the vital functions. Whenever coma prevails and respiration, the cardiovascular system, fluid and electrolyte balance, the renal system and other vital functions are at peril, intensive care is necessary and thus very few patients who reach the ward alive should ultimately succumb.

Gastric lavage is usually performed in the receiving ward. If there is any impairment of consciousness the airway must always be secured first with a cuffed endotracheal tube because of the danger of regurgitation or vomiting with inhalation. Frequently, if the drug has been taken more than four hours before admission no useful amount will appear in the gastric washings, but quantities of aspirin, barbiturates and tricyclic antidepressants, all commonly abused drugs, can sometimes be removed after eight or ten hours. This may also be the case when the patient is deeply unconscious and the intestine is relatively immobile. Some of the washings are sent to the laboratory for identification, and a sample is kept refrigerated should it be needed for forensic purposes.

If the patient is conscious lavage can be carried out without passage of an endotracheal tube provided the patient is lying on his left side in a head-down position. This procedure is decidedly unpleasant for the conscious patient and it may be difficult to obtain full co-operation.

When corrosive liquids such as caustic soda have been swallowed gastric lavage should not be attempted as it may lead to perforation of the oesophagus or stomach with the stomach tube.

Warm tap water is used for gastric lavage except in infants, when saline is used. The lavage should continue until the washings are clear. If the poison is Paraquat a quantity of Fuller's Earth (Bentonite) is introduced into the stomach before removing the tube. This treatment is combined with the administration of magnesium sulphate to produce a purgative action. This metabolically inert substance can absorb any Paraquat with which it may come into contact in its passage through the intestine, making the poison unavailable for absorption.

Specific antidotes

Whenever there is analytical confirmation or signs in an unconscious patient with respiratory depression that narcotics are responsible (e.g. 'pin-point' pupils) then naloxone (Narcan) should be promptly administered. The dose is initially 0.4 mg intravenously, and 0.8 mg repeated by the same route three minutes later. If there is no immediate response, with lightening of coma and improved ventilation, then the original diagnosis should be reconsidered. One dose of this antidote usually has an effect for only about four hours and, since the primary poison may be more prolonged in its action, more naloxone may be needed at intervals and in doses as indicated by the clinical state.

The effect of cyanide is usually so rapid that, in severe cases, the antidote cobalt edetate, which chelates (i.e. binds) the cyanide to render it inactive, should be given immediately in 40 ml of solution intravenously over the course of about one minute. If there is no prompt recovery another dose of 300 mg is indicated. Another treatment is sodium thiosulphate (25 ml of 50 % solution) given intravenously, converting cyanide to thiocyanate. Artificial ventilation should be with 100 % oxygen but direct expired air techniques should not be used because of the risk to the rescuer. The possibility of cyanide poisoning should be considered in all patients in the ICU who are being treated with sodium nitroprusside infusions. Each molecule of sodium nitroprusside is broken down in the body into five free cyanide radicals. One of these is trapped in the form of cyanmethaemoglobin leaving the other four radicals free to exert toxicity. Hydroxocobalamin (vitamin B_{12a}) may be used to prevent toxicity of cyanide liberated from sodium nitroprusside as it combines with cyanide to form cyanocobalamin. The disadvantage is that enormous doses are required.

Similarly, paracetamol overdose demands early, if not quite so immediate, attention because the antidotes are unavailing after about ten hours have elapsed since ingestion. At this stage the patient is commonly alert, responsive and with minimal symptoms. So a first dose of 2.5 g methionine should be given orally, followed by three similar doses at four-hourly intervals. If vomiting is a complication, the alternative is n-acetylcysteine, 150 mg/kg body weight given intravenously over 15 minutes, followed by an infusion of 50 mg/kg in 500 ml 5 % dextrose at 4, 8 and 12 hours. Advisedly, the patient should be kept under subsequent observation in the ICU to check for the development of hepatic failure and, if this does not arise, should be treated by the accepted regime (Chapter 5). Cysteamine (Mercaptamine) shows promise in the treatment of paracetamol poisoning which causes liver failure. This substance absorbs the toxic metabolite of paracetamol which causes the liver damage rendering it harmless, if given early enough. Mercaptamine is available from only some Poisons Centres.

Poisoning from the swallowing of iron salt preparations is seen more often in children. This requires gastric lavage with a 0.2 % aqueous solution of desferrioxamine, after which 10 g in 50 ml water should be left in the stomach. In addition, an intramuscular injection of 2 g in 10 ml water for an adult (1 g in 5 ml for a child) should be given, followed by an intravenous infusion of no more than 15 mg/kg/h, with a maximum of 80 mg/kg in 24 hours. Nevertheless, diarrhoea, shock and encephalopathy may supervene, especially if there has been any delay with this specific therapy. It is prudent, therefore, to admit any such patient to an ICU where the appropriate but active conservative management of these eventualities may be marshalled.

Among the other heavy elements, the effects of arsenic can be counteracted by dimercaprol, copper by d-penicillamine and mercury by n-acetylpenicillamine. In all such cases acute diarrhoea with water and electrolyte depletion may be a feature, demanding intensive therapy to correct this state.

In instances of drinking methanol, or ethylene glycol, the principle danger is of metabolic acidosis due to the enzymatic formation of formaldehyde and formic acid. This can be inhibited by infusing 50 % ethanol intravenously at the rate of 0.5 mg/kg every two hours for some days, this agent acting as a competitive substrate for the enzyme. At the same time any acidosis should be corrected by an infusion of sodium bicarbonate. Nevertheless, haemodialysis may become imperative in severe cases and patients who have taken these compounds are candidates for intensive care.

Poisoning by organophosphorus insecticides is not often encountered but is always potentially dangerous. The cholinergic manifestation of these compounds can be arrested by giving atropine by injection, in large (2 mg) and repeated doses, until a picture of marked 'atropinisation' is attained. Within the first 12–24 hours, moreover, the cholinergic-binding effect of the pesticide chemical may be reversed by giving pralidoxime in 2–3 ml water intramuscularly, or 6–20 ml intravenously, up to a total of three doses. In addition to this specific approach intensive care of a more general nature may be indispensible, to see that the patient is kept at complete rest, that any dehydration is corrected and, especially, to maintain a clear airway, sucking out excessive secretions and sometimes applying mechanical ventilation of the lungs.

Elimination of the toxin

Emptying the stomach, either by gastric aspiration and lavage or by induced emesis, normally comes within the province of the Accident and Emergency department. In the realm of intensive ward care, however, it may occasionally be expedient to consider some means of active intervention to hasten elimination of the toxin wherever the patient is seriously overdosed and where recovery is not being achieved by intensive conservative measures. Manoeuvres to this end should never be routinely or unselectively employed and, in fact, are applicable only in particular circumstances.

Forced diuresis

This form of treatment, contrary to popular belief, has a very limited application because few drugs are significantly excreted in the unchanged form. The majority of drugs are extensively detoxified by the liver. Inactive metabolites are excreted in the urine but liver metabolism can produce pharmacologically active metabolites.

The recognised complications of forced diuresis are pulmonary oedema, water intoxication, cerebral oedema, electrolyte and acid-base disturbances. Forced diuresis should never be undertaken lightly, as it is potentially lethal in elderly patients and in those with cardiac and renal disease. In practice, forced diuresis can be used in treatment of overdoses of salicylate, phenobarbitone and barbitone only. It has no place for other drugs and especially not for other forms of barbiturates. Salicylate, phenobarbitone and barbitone are all weak acids and tend to be more highly ionised in an alkaline environment. Thus, if the contents of the renal tubule are kept alkaline the reabsorption of the intact lipid-soluble molecule will be decreased and so excretion will be augmented. Besides, if the drug level in the tubule is low then the concentration gradient contributing to reabsorption will be reduced and excretion will tend to be enhanced.

Forced alkaline diuresis. This is indicated when the plasma levels of the following drugs are measured: phenobarbitone (100 mg/l); barbitone (100 mg/l); salicylates (500 mg/l). However, the clinical state of the patient must be considered in addition to the plasma drug levels.

The major complications of forced alkaline diuresis are those of fluid overload and electrolyte disturbance. Contra-indications are shock, impaired renal function and heart failure.

The procedure of forced alkaline diuresis may be hazardous and is therefore best conducted in an ICU. The baseline measurements used are electrolyte, arterial and urinary pH, blood sugar and drug levels.

Procedure for forced alkaline diuresis

1 Set up an IV infusion, a CVP line and a urinary catheter.

2 Give 20 mg frusemide intravenously.

3 In the first hour give:
   500 ml of 5% dextrose
   500 ml of 1.2% sodium bicarbonate ($NaHCO_3$)
   500 ml of 5% dextrose

4 Measure the urine flow at one hour.

5 If the urine flow is *more than* 3 ml/min continue the infusion with the dextrose/$NaHCO_3$ solutions to maintain a urine flow of 500 ml/hour.
   (a) The amount of $NaHCO_3$ should be adjusted to maintain a urinary pH 7.5–8.5.
   (b) Bolus doses of 30 mg frusemide IV may be necessary to achieve the correct urine flow level.
   (c) 10–20 mmol potassium (K^+) per litre of infused fluid should be given.

6 If the urine flow is *less than* 3 ml/min, this regime should be dicontinued.

Some ICUs prefer a more concentrated 8.4% $NaHCO_3$. This involves greater attention being given to the plasma electrolytes, especially sodium, given in this way.

Dialysis

Critical studies have indicated that the efficacy of dialysis in removing an excess of toxin from the body is often disappointing. Of course, such dialysis must be involved whenever renal failure enters as a complication of poisoning. Otherwise, while haemodialysis may be useful for treating overdoses of phenobarbitone and salicylates, forced alkaline diuresis is usually preferred as long as renal function is preserved. Peritoneal dialysis still has a place for the care of patients poisoned with lithium salts, ethylene glycol and sodium chlorate.

Both peritoneal dialysis and haemodialysis can be used to remove water-soluble poisons (Table 6.1). The technique is the same as in the treatment of acute renal failure and the same dialysing solutions are employed. Haemodialysis is more efficient but is usually discontinued after six to ten hours for logistic reasons. Peritoneal dialysis is more simple, requires less skill, can be used continuously and, because it causes a substantial loss of protein (about 1 g per cycle), clears small amounts of protein-bound drug as well as substances in free solution. The protein loss must be made good by giving intravenous plasma to prevent hypo-albuminaemia. It is emphasised that peritoneal dialysis often causes vomiting when used in patients whose consciousness is impaired so the stomach must be left empty or the airway secured when using this form of treatment. Peritoneal dialysis is sometimes limited to those poisoned with lithium salts and ethylene glycol.

Table 6.1 Dialysable and non-dialysable poisons

Dialysable poisons	
barbiturates	paraldehyde
salicylates	chloral hydrate
glutethimide (Doriden)	methaqualone
phenacetin	sodium chlorate
ethyl alcohol	boric acid
methyl alcohol	primidone
ethylene glycol (antifreeze)	sodium
thiocyanate	potassium
diphenylhydantoin	lithium
Non-dialysable poisons	
imipramine (Tofranil)	tranylcypromine (Parnate)
amitriptyline (Tryptizol)	pargyline
phenelzine (Nardil)	digoxin
chlordiazepoxide (Librium)	atropine
diazepam (Valium)	carbon tetrachloride

Haemoperfusion

The property of charcoal to absorb certain drugs and toxins has been known for many years. In 1964 the technique of haemoperfusion was introduced. The idea was to pass the patient's blood through a column of charcoal (the 'charcoal liver') and hence to remove the drug. There were considerable problems in the early stages with thrombocytopenia, leucopenia, emboli and pyrogen reactions. The new charcoal columns, in which the charcoal surface has been coated with a thin layer of biocompatible polymer, have overcome these difficulties. Damage to the blood passing over the charcoal is reduced and the elution of tiny particles of carbon into the blood is prevented. An acrylic hydrogel from which many soft contact lenses are made has been successfully used to coat charcoal in this way.

The haemoperfusion circuit is shown in the diagram (Fig. 6.1). The patient is connected to the circuit by an A-V shunt usually inserted in the forearm. Several different types of column are now available. A Watson-Marlow pump is used to produce an upward flow through the column of 200 ml/min. The patient is heparinised during the procedure. Frequent blood samples are taken to measure the plasma drug concentration, the platelet count and the heparin levels. The heparinisation is reversed with protamine sulphate at the end of the haemoperfusion; the duration of the procedure will depend on the drug concerned. The amount of drug removed can be calculated from the A-V plasma drug concentrations and the column flow rate.

Criteria for haemoperfusion. Haemoperfusion has been shown to be effective for barbiturate, glutethimide, methaqualone, salicylate, ethchlorvynol, meprobamate and theophylline poisoning. There are dangers attached to its use, principally those of bleeding during the heparinisation and for this reason criteria for haemoperfusion have been

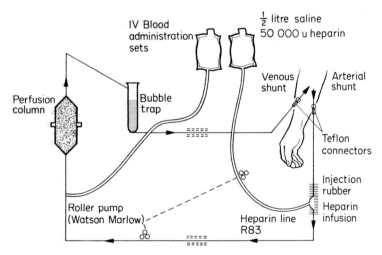

Fig. 6.1 A diagram of the set-up for haemoperfusion

established which are set out below. It is suggested that haemoperfusion should not be embarked upon unless three of the criteria are met:

1 severe clinical intoxication (i.e. the patient is unconscious with no responses at all), hypotension, hypothermia and hypoventilation;
2 progressive clinical deterioration despite good supportive management;
3 no evidence of improvement despite full resuscitation measures;
4 prolonged coma with added complications, e.g. pneumonia, chronic respiratory disease;
5 high plasma levels (mg/l) of the following drugs:

phenobarbitone	100
barbitone	100
other barbiturates	50
glutethimide	40
methaqualone	40
ethchlorvynol	150
meprobamate	100
trichlorethanol derivatives	50
salicylates	800

Results of haemoperfusion. Haemoperfusion has been shown to be effective in the management of patients with barbiturate and related hypnotic drug poisoning who were severely intoxicated and had high plasma drug concentrations. Studies have compared patients who met the criteria but were treated supportively and those who were haemoperfused. The latter group had a significantly lower mortality. The haemoperfusion reduced the duration of coma and the severity of respiratory complications. For drugs with large distribution volumes, such as tricyclic antidepressants, haemoperfusion is not of clinical benefit because only small amounts of the active drug are removed. Haemoperfusion has also been used in the management of serious Paraquat poisoning. Unfortunately it has made no impact on the eventual outcome and is now rarely used to treat such patients. In the future it seems that haemoperfusion may play a part in the management of serious paracetamol overdose when early treatment has been delayed, and in the growing problem of theophylline overdose.

Snake bites

The only naturally occuring venomous snake in Great Britain is the adder (*Vipera berus*). Fortunately severe poisoning is uncommon because the presence of a bite does not necessarily mean that venom has been injected. Poisoning may be recognised by persistent hypotension and polymorphonuclear leucocytosis. Bleeding may also be a feature, for example from the wound and injection sites, the gut and the kidney. Renal failure can occur. Treatment is symptomatic but severely-affected patients require Zagref antivenom which is a highly refined preparation and free of the side-effects of earlier preparations. Antivenom is given if hypotension persists, leucocytosis is present, there is metabolic acidosis or T-wave inversion on the ECG.

The majority of venomous snake bites in the United States are due to the pit viper family (*Crotalidae*) which includes the rattlesnake, copperhead and water moccasin.

The National Poisons Information Service

This service provides advice on poisonous substances and their treatment. A physician is available on call at each centre to provide additional information and to discuss management of the poisoned patient with the patient's doctor.

Telephone numbers of the five centres can be found in Appendix VII on page 240.

7

The Nervous System

The principal function of the nervous system is to convey information from one site to another and to integrate the activities of the several parts of the body. In man, the pathways taken are complex and co-ordination is obtained by complicated cross-connections.

The nervous system can be divided into the *central nervous system* (CNS) consisting of the brain and spinal cord, and the *peripheral nervous system* consisting of cranial and spinal nerves.

The brain

The brain is the largest part of the nervous system and is the expanded anterior part of the spinal cord. The various parts will be described.

The cerebral cortex. This makes up the greater part of the brain and comprises surface grey matter and deeper white matter. The *grey matter* is composed of nerve cells while the *white matter* is made up of the tracts of nerve fibres. The cerebral cortex consists of two cerebral hemispheres which contain the nerve cells and comprise the sensory and motor areas. In general, the right side of the brain controls the left side of the body, and *vice versa*. In addition, there are areas responsible for speech, hearing, vision, smell, learning and personality. The site of the complex processes of intelligence and insight is in the cerebral cortex. Spontaneous electrical potentials are emitted from the cerebral cortex. These can be amplified and recorded as an electro-encephalogram (EEG).

Electro-encephalography. The waveforms produced on the electro-encephalogram (EEG) can generally be classified according to their size and frequency. The alpha waves (at a frequency of 8 to 13 per second) are the predominant pattern in the adult, while slow delta waves (less than 4 per second) are predominant in children. These are also present during sleep as large, slow waves interspersed between bursts of 14 per second wave activity. Theta waves are slightly faster than the delta waves, but the fastest are the beta waves (Fig. 7.1).

The EEG can be of value in assessing the extent of brain damage, and also the prognosis; abnormal patterns may be a guide, while a straight-line tracing may indicate an irreversibly damaged brain. Before this situation is accepted, different EEG tracings showing similar patterns must be obtained, and other tests should be performed (page 158). Continuous EEG monitoring provides a non-invasive measurement of cerebral function that can be performed in paralysed ventilated patients.

The EEG can provide some localisation of pathological processes at a relatively low cost. Recently, the introduction of computer assisted processing and displaying of EEG information has improved its clinical usefulness. Recent interest in monitoring cerebral function in man centres on cortical and sub-cortical evoked responses (ER). An appropriate stimulus is applied to a peripheral or a cranial nerve and the electrical propagation of this stimulus in the brainstem and cerebral cortex is recorded by means of scalp electrodes. Repeated stimuli and responses are electronically stored and processed; cerebral and brain stem dysfunction can be monitored in this way and the technique is useful in assessing the progress or remission of CNS disorders.

The cerebellum. The functions of this part of the brain have been deduced from animal experiments and from symptoms in patients suffering from cerebellar disease. These symptoms include unsteadiness, incoordination, nystagmus, disordered movements and tremor. It can be assumed that the cerebellar nuclei are involved in balance, posture, equilibration and the intensity and distribution of muscle tone.

The pons. This bundle of fibres carries impulses from one side of the cerebellum to the other, co-ordinating muscle movements on both sides of the body.

The thalamus. This is a station in the sensory pathways to the cerebral cortex. Fibres from the spinal cord and lower parts of the brain form synapses with other neurones going to the sensory cortex. Lesions of the thalamus may produce pain.

The hypothalamus. Situated in the floor of the third ventricle, the hypothalamus is concerned with temperature control, water balance, carbohydrate and fat metabolism, blood pressure and sleep.

The reticular activating system. This is associated with awareness and consciousness. It is a collection of scattered nerve cells in relation to the central canal and aqueduct. It reaches from the medulla to the thalamus.

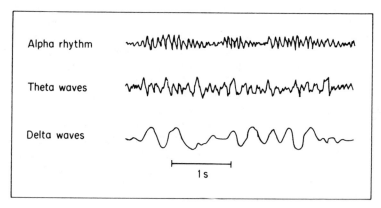

Fig. 7.1 Different types of EEG waves

The motor system. This is composed of the motor cortex and the *pyramidal tract* fibres, which pass down through the internal capsule and cerebral peduncles to the anterior horn cells of the spinal cord. Most fibres cross to the other side, but some remain uncrossed. The motor neurones then pass from the anterior horn cells to the muscle fibres.

In addition to the pyramidal tract, there is the *extra-pyramidal system*, which is also concerned with movement. This system has complex connections with the cerebellum, vestibular system and the sub-cortical nuclei. Disease of this system may produce Parkinsonism, which is characterised by rigidity, tremor, lack of facial expression and slow muscular movements.

The junction between the muscle fibre and the terminal axon of the motor neurone is called the neuromuscular or myoneural junction (Fig. 7.2). The chemical transmitter acetylcholine is synthesised from choline and acetyl co-enzyme A within the nerve terminals. The terminal axon is rich in mitrochondria which supply energy for the formation of acetyl co-enzyme A and in synaptic vesicles which store the acetylcholine. Acetylcholine is released from the vesicles when a sufficiently strong nerve impulse reaches the nerve terminals, and diffuses across the synaptic cleft to reach the receptors on the motor end-plate to achieve depolarisation. This chemical event is followed by muscle contraction, a mechanical event

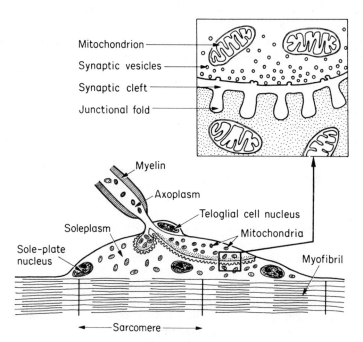

Fig. 7.2 Diagram of a motor end-plate on a muscle fibre, longitudinal section

in the muscle fibre. Acetylcholine is broken down by acetylcholinesterase of the post-junctional membrane to produce choline and acetate. The choline is then available for transport back into the nerve terminals to be acetylated by acetyl co-enzyme A into acetylcholine again. Anticholinesterase drugs such as neostigmine (Prostigmin) prevent the interaction of cholinesterase and hence lead to increased local concentrations of acetylcholine.

It is important to understand this simplified explanation of neuromuscular transmissions in order to appreciate the action of muscle relaxant drugs, which block the receptor sites.

The sensory system. Stimulation of sensory receptors sends impulses up ascending pathways in the spinal cord to the sensory cortex. The receptors may be in the skin, muscle, tendons, joints or viscera. Chemoreceptors and baroreceptors are situated in the great vessels. Excitation of the sensory receptors may be by electrical, thermal, mechanical or chemical stimuli. There are receptors in the skin for pain, touch and temperature. Pain may also be visceral in origin and may be referred to a different site on the body surface which is innervated from the same segment of the spinal cord. This occurs in gall bladder disease when the pain may be felt at the shoulder tip.

Paraesthesiae. This is a term used to describe tingling without external stimuli. It may be due to disease of peripheral nerves.

Reflexes. These are responses of effector organs following stimulation of a receptor. The link is by a neurone arc, and can occur at spinal level. Examples include tendon jerks and pupillary reflexes.

Cranial nerves. These are twelve pairs of nerves primarily innervating sense organs, muscles and glands of the head and neck. The vagus (Xth) nerve is part of the autonomic system and innervates the internal organs of the chest and abdomen.

The autonomic nervous system. This involuntary motor system innervates the heart, lungs, digestive tract and other abdominal viscera. There are two complementary parts to this system:

1 *The sympathetic system.* This is characterised by adrenaline-type reactions, such as increased heart rate, dilated pupils, increased blood flow to muscles, peripheral vascoconstriction and 'goose flesh'.

2 *The parasympathetic system.* These fibres emerge with some cranial nerves. The most important part of this system is the vagus with its major action on heart, lungs and intestinal tract. Characteristic parasympathetic vagal effects are slowing of the heart and increased secretions.

Cerebrospinal fluid. The brain and spinal cord are bathed in a clear, colourless fluid—the cerebrospinal fluid (CSF). This is secreted into the ventricles and subarachnoid space by the choroid plexus. The fluid circulates through the ventricles and over the surface of the brain and maintains a constant pressure and environment around the brain and spinal cord. The constituents and pressure of the cerebrospinal fluid will be altered by subarachnoid haemorrhage, brain tumour and meningitis. Blood in the CSF is a serious sign commonly caused by subarachnoid haemorrhage or trauma.

The pressure of the CSF can be measured by connecting a manometer tube to the hub of the needle at lumbar puncture. The normal pressure is 10–13 cmH$_2$O(100–130 mmCSF). Obstruction to the circulation of the CSF, whether by space-occupying lesions or cerebral oedema (page 151), will produce a rise in intracranial pressure (ICP) and a high CSF pressure. When the outflow of CSF from the ventricles is obstructed, *internal hydrocephalus* is produced. The raised pressure will tend to push down the cerebellum and medulla into the foramen magnum at the base of the skull. This serious condition is known as *pressure cone* or 'coning'. Headache, vomiting and papilloedema are signs of raised intracranial pressure.

Investigations employed for the detection of space-occupying lesions of the brain, such as tumours or blood clots, detect distortion of the normal anatomy. These include:

(a) *Angiography*. Contrast media injected into the carotid or vertebral arteries will show abnormal circulation or distortions of the normal vascular pattern.

(b) *Ventriculography*. Air or radio-opaque dye will outline the ventricular system and demonstrate distortion or blockage.

(c) *Echo-encephalography*. Using an ultrasonic source, high frequency waves can be reflected from tumours, haematomas or bony structures and displayed on a cathode ray tube. By this means, mid-line shift and space-occupying lesions may be detected.

(d) *Computerised axial tomography (CAT) scanning*. Radiographic examination of the brain presents a special problem because of the very high density of the bones of the skull. The basic radiograph is an image of the entire part being X-rayed so that structures of varying density through that body area are superimposed on each other. The *tomograph* consists of a radiograph visualising just a horizontal view of the area in question with the overlaying and underlying structures blurred out. This is achieved by using a moving X-ray source and photographic plate.

The development of a technique called computerised axial tomography has played a major advance in diagnosis. This new technique takes pictures as a series of tomographic sections. The head of the patient is scanned by a fan beam of X-rays. The X-ray tube and the X-ray detectors are fitted to a common frame so that the X-rays passing through the patient are detected by the sensory devices which consist of crystals of sodium iodide. These crystals emit a 'blip' of light when they receive the radiation and the 'blips' of light are counted up by electronic means. The X-ray tube and detector make repeated transverse scans of the skull but each time in a slightly different plane. Each scan takes less than a minute and a complete examination takes about 30 minutes. A computer controls the mechanism and processes the readings so that complete sets of pictures are built up. The total radiation dose for a series of scans is comparable to that for a single plain film radiograph covering the same area. CAT scanning has the advantage that it is non-invasive and without hazards or discomfort to the patient. Very restless patients or small children who cannot keep still for the brief time required to conduct the examination may need to be anaesthetised.

Central nervous system disorders

Those requiring intensive care are usually conditions in which the brain has been damaged or depressed by one of the following:

(a) *Trauma*—contusion or destruction of brain tissue with or without skull fracture.
(b) *Vascular disorders*—haemorrhage, thrombosis, hypertensive encephalopathy, circulatory failure.
(c) *Poisons*—barbiturates, narcotics, tranquillisers, alcohol etc.
(d) *Hypoxia*—after cardiac arrest, suffocation, carbon monoxide poisoning, respiratory failure.
(e) *Space occupying lesions*—tumours, abscess.
(f) *Endocrine disorders*—diabetes, myxoedema, Addison's disease.
(g) *Miscellaneous*—hypothermia, hypercarbia, epilepsy, electrolyte disturbances, infection etc.

Brain damage may in turn produce one or more of the following effects all of which must be treated at the same time as the cause:

1 Unconsciousness
2 Convulsions
3 Cerebral oedema
4 Respiratory failure of central origin

The basic treatment of severe disorders of the central nervous system revolves around the treatment of these four conditions. Note that several important factors relating to the intercranial pressure need to be considered before treatment; these are illustrated in the ICP triad (Fig. 7.3).

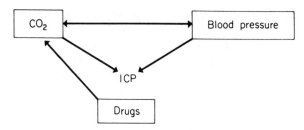

Fig. 7.3 The intracranial pressure triad emphasises the need to consider the Pa_{CO_2}, blood pressure and drugs administered to patients with raised ICP

1 Consciousness and unconsciousness

Many of the neurological disturbances dealt with in the intensive care unit are disturbances of consciousness, which is defined as awareness of and attention to the surroundings and depends upon the activity of the reticular activating system (RAS) which stretches from the medulla to the third ventricle. There are many connections to this system, particularly from the sensory system and especially from pain endings.

Disturbances in the activity of the RAS produce disturbances in the level of consciousness such that protective reflexes may be reduced or abolished. The degree of unconsciousness may vary from light levels where the patient may be roused (stupor), to deep coma which usually leads to death. *Coma* is defined as not obeying commands, not opening the eyes and not uttering any words. Any of the causes of brain damage (see page 140) may result in unconsciousness. The severity of that damage will determine the degree of unconsciousness. Minor disturbances will result only in drowsiness, restlessness and disorientation. However, deterioration may be progressive and require urgent treatment. At the other end of the scale, deep coma with absent reflexes may occur. Here the outcome is invariably fatal.

Head injuries. The care of patients admitted to hospital following head injury places a considerable strain on the available resources of the National Health Service. They account for about 10 % of all new cases presenting to Accident and Emergency Departments. Most of these cases are mild and two-thirds are discharged within 48 hours, but 70 % of deaths from road traffic accidents are due to head injuries. It is thought that about 1200 brain-damaged survivors leave hospitals in England and Wales every year, their average age being about 30 years; half of them will probably never work again. In England and Wales in 1972, 60 % of deaths ascribable to head injury occurred before the victim could be admitted to hospital. There is now good evidence that secondary brain damage is commonly suffered by head-injured patients in hospital and that an appreciable proportion of the death and morbidity attributable to head injury is due to potentially preventable events. Criteria for admission of patients following head injury vary between hospitals.

It is desirable that any patient who has had an injury severe enough to cause concussion is admitted to hospital for a period of observation. Management of patients with a head injury involves not only surgical treatment and nursing care of the unconscious patient, but also early recognition and treatment of any complications which may occur. It is to achieve this early recognition—particularly of the life-threatening extradural haematoma (Fig. 7.4)—that patients with apparently trivial injuries are admitted to hospital. A substantial number of patients with severe head injuries who reach hospital alive are hypoxic, hypotensive or anaemic, usually due to associated injuries.

Intracranial pressure (ICP)

Normal	1–10 mmHg (0.1–1.3 kPa)
Slightly increased	11–20 mmHg (1.5–2.7 kPa)
Moderately increased	21–40 mmHg (2.8–5.3 kPa)

Cerebral perfusion pressure (CPP)

$$CPP = \begin{bmatrix} \text{mean systemic} \\ \text{arterial pressure} \end{bmatrix} - \begin{bmatrix} \text{intracranial} \\ \text{pressure (ICP)} \end{bmatrix} = \begin{matrix} 80\,\text{mmHg} \\ (10.6\,\text{kPa}) \end{matrix}$$

Sometimes the jugular venous pressure is substituted for ICP.

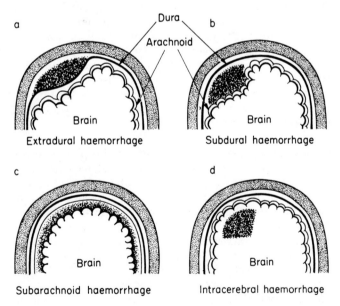

Fig. 7.4 Bleeding within the skull; extradural, subdural, subarachnoid and intracerebral

Classification. Head-injured patients may be put into four categories as an aid to their management:

Group 1   patients who have a minimal disturbance of consciousness or a history of loss of consciousness;

Group 2   patients with moderate disturbance of consciousness, but without focal neurological deficit;

Group 3   patients with significant alteration of consciousness combined with appropriate response to painful stimuli and focal neurological deficit, and who cannot follow simple commands;

Group 4   comatose patients with obvious head injury.

The management of these patients is shown schematically in Fig. 7.5. Turning the head to one or other side causes large rises in ICP because of obstruction to blood flow down the jugular veins. Few head-injured patients require definitive neurological procedures. In the United

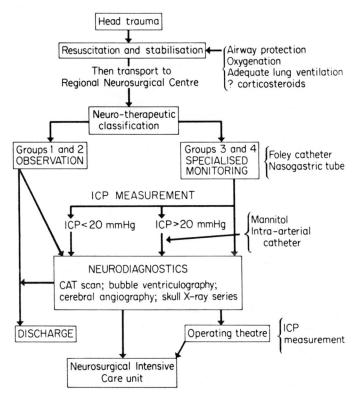

Fig. 7.5 The ideal disposition of head-injured patients

Kingdom 95 % of all patients admitted to hospital are managed outside neurosurgical units.

ICP monitoring. Many patients who are strongly suspected of having a significant elevation of ICP are, unfortunately, still treated without any attempt to measure that pressure and, therefore, with no hope of selecting optimal therapy and management to control it.

Figure 7.6 shows an ICP-volume curve, and is analogous to the pressure-volume relationship for the lungs discussed in Chapter 3. The reciprocal of compliance is elastance:

$$\text{elastance} = \frac{\text{pressure change observed}}{\text{volume change introduced}}$$

Suppose a small balloon is introduced through a small hole in the skull to lie within the extradural space. Also suppose that 1 ml of liquid is periodically injected into the balloon and the pressure produced inside the skull observed. In the region of low pressure elastance (Fig. 7.6) quite a large volume can be injected before the ICP begins to rise sharply. However, there comes a point ('breakpoint') after which each increment of fluid injected into the balloon produces a larger rise in ICP. When eventually the ICP equals the mean arterial pressure in the brain, then cerebral perfusion ceases. Unless ICP is measured, we do not know whether any given patient lies in the low elastance region or in the high elastance region. Patients in the low elastance region can tolerate more insults (such as further rises in ICP provoked by stimulation, e.g. suctioning) than those nearer cerebral death in the high elastance region.

ICP may be measured by placing a suitable sensor extradurally, subdurally or within one of the cerebral ventricles where the pressure of

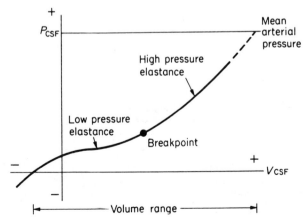

Fig. 7.6 The relationship between CSF pressure and volume within the skull

intraventricular fluid (IVF) is measured. Figure 7.7 shows an implanted extradural transducer and Fig. 7.8 shows an external transducer connected to a ventricular catheter. It is essential that all care is taken to avoid infection via these catheters and transducers. The IVF system has the advantage that CSF can be drained off to relieve pressure in an emergency. The continuous recording of ICP permits the recognition of significant trends and thus immediate medical or surgical intervention.

Clinical signs of raised ICP. An expanding intracranial lesion (such as bleeding within the skull) may lead to a vicious circle being set up of secondary factors which reduce the supply of oxygen to the brain. An expanding intracranial lesion, increasing cerebral oedema, and a rising ICP are aggravated by respiratory insufficiency, hypoxia, hypercapnia venous congestion, hypotension, anaemia and by certain anaesthetic drugs. The clinical signs of a rising ICP are:

(a) deterioration in the level of consciousness;
(b) progressive slowing of the pulse rate;
(c) a rising systolic blood pressure;
(d) increasing pulse pressure;
(e) a change in the respiratory pattern, which may become slow, irregular or periodic;
(f) Dilating or non-reacting pupils which may also be unequal.

The Glasgow Coma Scale. This is the best means for the intensive care nurse to record the neurological status of a head-injured patient (Fig. 7.9). This scale is clear and informative and avoids the use of confusing words

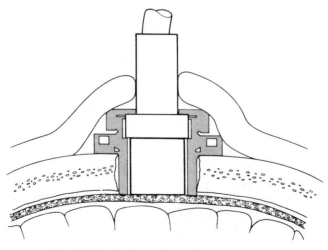

Fig. 7.7 An implanted extradural transducer

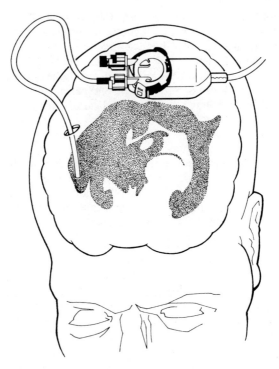

Fig. 7.8 An external transducer with ventricular catheter

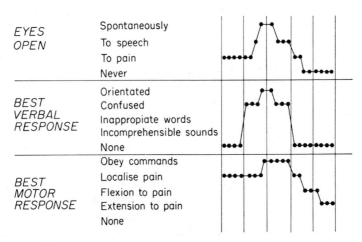

Fig. 7.9 The Glasgow Coma Scale

such as semiconscious, stupor or semicomatose. It depends on the observation and recording of the response to three separate aspects of behaviour—eye opening, verbal response, and the motor response to a verbal command or painful stimulus. The Glasgow Coma Scale does not record some basic criteria such as vital signs, pupillary size and reactivity, oculovestibular response, ICP, and lateralisation (movement and strength) of arms and legs. A composite chart is used to permit recording of these measurements in addition to the Coma Scale (Appendix VI). The additional observations relate to:

Eye signs. Pupil size and reaction may be a guide to the site and degree of brain damage, and must be recorded accurately. The time interval between the observations will depend upon the condition of the patient but a half hour is usually sufficient. For example, an extradural haemorrhage may result in a dilated pupil on the affected side which does not react to light directly or when the pupil on the other side is illuminated.

Vital signs. Pulse rate and rhythm, systolic and diastolic blood pressure, respiration and temperature must be charted and changes reported to the medical staff in charge of the patient. Signs of cerebral compression include a slow pulse rate, a rise in blood pressure, slowing of respiration leading to periodic respiration (*Cheyne-Stokes*) and apnoea. As the sequence proceeds, the pulse rate will increase and the blood pressure will fall. The situation may be aggravated by hypoxia due to airway obstruction. A rising pulse rate and blood pressure with rapid shallow respirations are associated with hypoxia.

There are two types of periodic breathing. The most common is '*Cheyne-Stokes breathing*' which is characterised by a slow waxing and waning of respiration followed by apnoea. Each cycle lasts 45 seconds to 3 minutes. As well as in lesions of the nervous system, it has been recorded in left ventricular failure and in narcotic poisoning. '*Biot's breathing*' is much less common. This form of periodic breathing has 'runs' of several breaths, say four or more at a time, followed suddenly by a period of complete cessation of respiration. Another normal series of breaths follows and the cycle repeats itself. The duration of the cycle is very variable (as short as 10 seconds or as long as one minute). It is found in meningitis, brain compression and brain destruction. Although hyperpyrexia is a late sign, the temperature may be normal or even low in neurological cases of the type under discussion.

Trends are the most important aspect of records in neurological cases. Early changes should be recorded and reported without delay, as surgical intervention may be required urgently.

Additional signs. These include headache, vomiting, irritability and neck stiffness. The latter may be due to blood in the CSF and can be confirmed by lumbar puncture. In head injury, blood or CSF may leak from the nose or ear. Papilloedema is evidence of raised ICP.

There is also an association between CNS diseases and ECG abnormalities which is thought to be mediated as abnormalities of the sympathetic tone to the heart. Increases in ICP may give rise to ECG changes such as prominent U waves, ST-T segment changes, notched P waves and shortening of Q-T intervals; prolongation of the Q-T interval is an ominous sign.

Excessive sympathetic activity following markedly raised ICP may lead to left ventricular strain and secondary pulmonary oedema.

Care of the unconscious patient. Attention must be directed to the following points:

(i) *Protection of the airway.* Laryngoscopy will show whether the reflexes of the pharynx and larynx are intact. If not, or if there is any doubt, the trachea must be intubated with a cuffed tube (page 80). The cuff should be inflated until there is no leak of gas from the trachea. If these measures are likely to be necessary for more than one week, tracheostomy may be required. In any case, intubation is usually performed as the emergency procedure followed by tracheostomy at a later date. Until the trachea can be protected by these means, the patient should be placed on his side in the semi-prone position with a slight head-down tilt. This will allow vomit and secretions to drain from the mouth. If contamination is suspected, bronchoscopy should be performed. Suction of the pharynx will, of course, be necessary prior to intubation for the same reason. All mechanical procedures within the pharynx, larynx and trachea (e.g. suction, laryngoscopy and intubation) are associated with *large rises in arterial pressure and intracranial pressure.* The patient should not be stimulated by suction catheters unless absolutely necessary. Doses of anaesthetic agents or beta-adrenergic receptor-blocking drugs may be required to attenuate these pressor responses in certain patients.

(ii) *Respiratory insufficiency.* Respiration may be severely depressed and measurements of blood gases, tidal and minute volumes will assist in making a decision regarding IPPV. If the patient has to be ventilated, care should be taken in the control of arterial $P\text{co}_2$. It is probably best to keep this as near to normal as possible, although hyperventilation may be used to aid in the management of the cerebral oedema in the first few days of treatment. If there is some breathing and underventilation is not severe enough for IPPV, oxygen may be added to the inspired air in order to raise the $P\text{o}_2$, bearing in mind that carbon dioxide accumulation may occur. The $P\text{co}_2$ level should be monitored.

(iii) *Circulatory insufficiency.* Hypotension must be corrected and blood replacement will be required following multiple injuries.

Intravenous fluids may be necessary bearing in mind that cerebral oedema should not be aggravated. The systolic blood pressure should not be allowed to fall below 80 mmHg (10.6 kPa). Systolic blood pressures of more than 160 mmHg (21.2 kPa) should be avoided because arterial hypertension in the presence of brain damage may lead to increased cerebral oedema. The hypertension due to hypoxia, pain, a full bladder, restlessness or an expanding brain lesion must be excluded before administering sedation, analgesics and antihypertensive treatment.

(iv) *Care of the eyes and skin.* Nursing care is required as detailed in Chapter 10.

(v) *Bladder.* The bladder will certainly require catheterisation and closed drainage. Fluid balance charts must be carefully kept.

(vi) *Prevention of infection.* Comatose patients are liable to infection and the lungs are particularly vulnerable. For this reason antibiotics are given prophylactically.

(vii) *Nutrition.* This aspect must not be neglected, and nutrition is best given by a nasogastric tube. The same principles apply as in Chapter 9. Intravenous feeding may have a limited place if there are large gastric aspirates after multiple injuries. Gastrointestinal bleeding in brain-injured patients may develop as a consequence of stress, therapy with corticosteroids or the presence of the nasogastric tube. Cimetidine or ranitidine, which block the secretion of acid from the stomach mucosa, is useful to prevent this complication.

(viii) *Sedation.* This should be avoided in order that the level of unconsciousness is not masked. However, an extremely restless patient may provoke dangerously large rises in ICP in the absence of sedation. It is very difficult to steer a course between these two requirements and no general recommendations can be made. Infusions of short-acting sedatives and/or the new non-depolarising muscle relaxants may be useful.

(ix) *Body temperature.* The development of *hyperthermia* is associated with serious metabolic problems and must be treated without delay at all costs. Vigorous application of iced water and ice in plastic bags over the surface of the body, especially in the axillae and groins (axillary and femoral arteries), should be used to reduce the temperature. Evaporation is assisted by the use of fans. Cooling is facilitated by promoting vasodilation, for instance by drugs such as diazepam. These drugs also help to abolish shivering; a muscle relaxant is useful if the patient is receiving passive IPPV of the lungs. Care should be taken that too low a body temperature is not produced ('overswing' or 'afterdrop') and treatment should be stopped when the rectal or nasopharyngeal temperature reaches 38°C. Axillary or peripheral temperature measurements are quite unreliable; core temperatures should always be taken.

2   Convulsions (fits)

Convulsions are involuntary uncoordinated contractions which may arise from one focus in the brain or may be generalised. They may occur as a result of brain damage. Convulsions are dangerous for several reasons:

(a) they interfere with normal respiration by preventing smooth, rhythmical, co-ordinated action of the respiratory muscles;

(b) they increase oxygen consumption and requirement by the immense amount of muscle activity;

(c) they damage the brain by the abnormal discharge of electrical activity;

(d) they may result in injury due to the violence of the convulsions and fractures may be produced.

The degree of damage depends upon the severity of the convulsions. Repeated attacks of hypoxia together with discharge of electrical activity from the brain cells both contribute to further mental deterioration.

Epilepsy. This is a term usually confined to convulsions from idiopathic causes. It can, however, be used in a more general way to describe fits due to trauma, tumours, vascular disturbances, and infections. Drugs and metabolic disturbances may give rise to epileptiform attacks. When the convulsions are continuous the condition is described as *status epilepticus*.

Treatment of convulsions. The basis of treatment is to cut down the abnormal activity of the brain and reduce its irritability. Barbiturates are particularly useful for this and phenobarbitone 200 mg can be given intravenously or intramuscularly if the situation is not urgent. An alternative is phenytoin 200 mg by the same route; care is necessary with the IV route in case the plasma calcium concentration is lowered. Phenytoin 50 mg IM can then be given 8-hourly to maintain control. Diazepam, too, is useful for this purpose. Phenytoin and phenobarbitone are also given as prophylactic drugs.

Status epilepticus is a much more serious condition which should be treated in the same way but using both the above drugs together if necessary. Cerebral hypoxia must be counteracted by giving oxygen by mask, but this may not markedly increase the oxygenation if the fits are not controlled. Thiopentone, Althesin or chlormethiazole, given as a continuous infusion, are useful methods of control and large doses of diazepam have also been used intravenously. The utmost care should be taken to ensure that the arterial pressure and hence the cerebral perfusion pressure is not depressed unduly. These drugs are preferable to paraldehyde. Full facilities for endotracheal intubation and ventilation of the lungs with oxygen must be available when these drugs are used. If this regime does not control the fits, IPPV must be instigated using muscle relaxants such as pancuronium to produce muscular paralysis. Although this will allow oxygenation and control convulsions, it must be remembered that the convulsive brain discharges are still present and these may cause brain damage even in the paralysed patient. For this reason diazepam should be given in addition to the muscle relaxants. The cause of the convulsions must also be treated remembering that fits should not be lightly labelled as idiopathic.

3 Cerebral oedema

The most important component of the so-called *blood-brain barrier* is the endothelial cells of the intracerebral capillaries, where tight junctions between adjacent cells present a permeability barrier which resists the passage of all but the smallest molecules into the brain and tissue CSF. To cross this barrier, drugs must be at least partially soluble in lipid. The barrier may be damaged and made permeable following CNS injuries and diseases. This damage may be manifest as 'leakage' of contrast medium into the brain after specialised X-ray examinations and clinically it is evident as cerebral oedema.

Cerebral oedema is a condition in which there is excess water in the tissues of the brain. Although the grey and white matter are taken as one, it is possible that the causes are different in each case. Whatever the cause of this condition, it is probably very complex. The following is the most probable explanation of excessive water occurring in the white matter. In normal tissues there is a finely balanced mechanism between the hydrostatic and osmotic pressures at the capillary end of the circulation. In the arterial part of the loop, fluid is pushed out hydrostatically against the osmotic pull in the opposite direction. The reverse is true at the venous end, where the hydrostatic pressure is less than the osmotic pressure. If this balance is disturbed so that the fluid is not reabsorbed, the result is excess fluid in the brain tissues. The causes fall into three groups:

(i) Reduced osmotic pressure
(ii) Capillary endothelial damage
(iii) Disturbance of venous drainage

Although the osmotic pressure may be reduced by starvation, the latter two groups are the most important. The capillary permeability can be altered by hypoxia, drugs and toxins, infections and electrolyte disturbances. This will allow the passage of large molecules as well as sodium and chloride. Tumours and brain trauma may disturb the venous circulation.

The increase in bulk will exert pressure effects as there is little room for expansion in the rigid skull. The first effect will be on the blood vessels and CSF. As the pressure builds up, ischaemia will be produced. If the cause is unilateral there will be a shift of the brain across the mid-line. Pressure on the reticular activating system will result in unconsciousness; in addition, the vital centres will be damaged resulting in pulse, blood pressure and respiratory disturbances. A fall in pulse rate is accompanied by a rise in blood pressure in many cases.

Treatment. This is directed to removing excess fluid at the venous end of the capillary loop, and is based on the intravenous use of hypertonic solutions which do not easily pass across the 'blood-brain barrier'. At the same time fluid restriction is advisable. Treatment of the cause, such as hypoxia or infection, is obviously required.

The hypertonic solutions will produce a diuresis and the unconscious patient will require catheterisation. The increase in blood volume produced by these solutions often causes an increase in bleeding. Unfortunately, as they pass into the brain further oedema and swelling will occur and this 'rebound' may reduce their effectiveness.

Mannitol. This is the most effective of the intravenous solutions available at present and is best given as a 20 % preparation in saline. Gentle warming may be necessary to dissolve crystals still present in the supersaturated solution. Being a sugar it is non-toxic and maintains renal flow. The dose is 0.5–1.0 g/kg body weight given 4–6-hourly for up to 24–48 hours although smaller doses given more often are preferred in some ICUs. Urine output must be closely monitored. If the renal excretion of mannitol does not occur in the normal manner there is a risk of renal tubular necrosis. Plasma osmolarity is normally 285 ± 6 mOsmol/l. If blood osmolarity is greater than 310 mOsmol/l mannitol enters the brain and, therefore, the effect of the drug is defeated. However, there is less 'rebound' with mannitol than other solutions. Rebound is the secondary increase in brain water if the drug is not properly excreted by the kidneys. Urea, triple strength plasma, 25 % saline and 50 % sucrose are not used now because they readily pass into the brain and cause rebound.

Dexamethasone. This steroid probably acts by restoring the integrity of the 'blood-brain barrier' and may also facilitate the conversion of lactic acid to glucose and thereby reduce intracerebral acidosis. There is less salt and water retention than with other steroids but its action is necessarily slow. The usual regime is to give 8 mg IV and follow this with 4 mg IM 6-hourly. As the patient improves, the dosage can be reduced over about 5 days. Although dexamethasone is effective in combating the oedema associated with cerebral tumours (notably gliomas) it is of much less value in other states. The place of dexamethasone and the other corticosteroids in the treatment of head injuries has not yet been resolved.

Lasix (frusemide). Excess water can be removed from the body by the diuretic action of frusemide. The usual dose is 1 mg/kg body weight by intravenous or intramuscular injection. Frusemide may also be of value if given before the administration of osmotic dehydration agents (e.g. mannitol) to prevent adverse effects from circulatory overload.

There are two other methods in which brain swelling may be reduced. These are controlled hyperventilation and hypothermia. They both depend upon reduction of blood flow for their effect.

Controlled hyperventilation. Ventilation of the lungs in excess of the normal minute volume will reduce the Pa_{CO_2}. The result of this is cerebral vasoconstriction which reduces the cerebral blood flow particularly when the Pa_{CO_2} is below 25 mmHg (3.3 kPa). This limit of Pa_{CO_2} reduction should not be exceeded. The benefits of Pa_{CO_2} reduction, if any, last only a few days. However, Pa_{CO_2} should not be allowed to rise above the mean of the normal range, 40 mmHg (5.3 kPa).

Hypothermia. The value of hypothermia is not universally accepted although experimental work shows that it reduces intracranial pressure and cerebral oedema.

Hyperbaric oxygen probably has no use in the treatment of cerebral oedema even though hypoxia was the original cause.

4 Respiratory failure

This is a common sequel to brain damage and may require IPPV if there is severe underventilation. IPPV may be indicated for other reasons such as cerebral oedema.

The advantages of controlled ventilation in head-injured patients are:

(a) ICP is reduced; also the effects of cerebral oedema are reduced;
(b) there is usually an improvement in arterial oxygenation;
(c) exhausting overbreathing is relieved;
(d) convulsions and decerebrate spasm are controlled;
(e) body temperature is more easily controlled.

Hypocapnia may be instituted when:

(i) ICP exceeds 30 mmHg (4.0 kPa) despite other measures;
(ii) convulsions and decerebrate spasms cannot be controlled;
(iii) the Pa_{O_2} is less than 70 mmHg (9.3 kPa) and does not improve with increase in the inspired oxygen concentration.

Peripheral nervous system disorders

Disorders of peripheral motor nerves may require treatment in the ICU particularly if they present a threat to breathing. In cases of poliomyelitis, polyneuritis and myasthenia gravis, there is lack of motor activity. Here, IPPV may be essential when respiratory failure is clinically present or threatened. The decision to ventilate should not be delayed in these cases until blood gas results are available. An arterial blood sample should be taken before ventilation is begun. 'Fits' may also interfere with breathing to such an extent that artificial ventilation is required. Tetanus and strychnine poisoning are instances of this and here full muscle paralysis is required combined with IPPV.

Acute poliomyelitis

Until a few years ago, poliomyelitis was the commonest single condition in which artificial respiration was needed for long periods. Poliomyelitis is a virus infection of the anterior horn cells of the spinal cord, producing weakness or paralysis. If the intercostal muscles and diaphragm are affected respiratory failure may result (*spinal poliomyelitis*). Medullary centres and cranial nerve nuclei may be affected if the disease involves the brain stem (*bulbar poliomyelitis*). Dysphagia, laryngeal and pharyngeal paralysis may result leading to aspiration of food and secretions. The disease may be mixed (spinal and bulbar) in some patients.

Isolation is essential in a special unit, the disease being infectious. Although the disease would not be treated in a general ICU, the treatment involves intensive care principles. Attention is directed towards:

    (i) prevention of aspiration of vomit and secretions;

    (ii) respiratory support.

Emergency procedures involve endotracheal intubation with a cuffed tube. Tracheostomy will be required if there is respiratory involvement. In cases with bulbar involvement (where there is paralysis of the muscles of swallowing) there is danger of secretions in the mouth spilling over into the lungs; a cuffed tube is essential in such cases even if a tank (iron lung) respirator is used. Efficient suction is mandatory in wet cases. A sign of respiratory failure in these cases is rapid shallow breathing, often with a truncated or 'cut-off' pattern. The blood pressure may rise and tachycardia may be present. Vital capacity measurements may be useful in difficult cases and reductions to 30% of normal would require ventilation. Ventilation with an Ambu bag should be carried out until the patient can be mechanically ventilated. The type of ventilator would depend on the routine of the unit, but tank ventilators still have a place in poliomyelitis units.

Polyneuritis

This is a composite term for what is really a group of similar diseases (acute toxic polyneuritis, infective neuronitis and Guillian Barré syndrome). Diffuse injury of the peripheral parts of the lower motor and sensory neurones can be produced. It can accompany any infection both acute (e.g. diphtheria) and chronic (e.g. tuberculosis), and can occur as an acute infective process of viral origin. Diabetes, vitamin deficiencies and poisons may produce a similar picture. It usually affects limb muscles, but may occasionally involve intercostal muscles and the diaphragm. Respiration will then require urgent support with IPPV. Any obvious cause must be found and treated, but lung ventilation may be required for some considerable time as virtually complete recovery is usual.

Myasthenia gravis

This is a chronic disease characterised by variable factors and weakness of voluntary muscles which gradually recover with rest. It is a condition in which there is interference with transmission at the neuromuscular junction (Fig. 7.2). In some ways, it is similar to the block produced by the non-depolarising muscle relaxants such as tubocurarine. There is probably an abnormality in the response of the motor end-plate to the action of acetylcholine. The clinical picture is that of muscle weakness and fatigue. At the time of admission, the patient's respiratory function should be assessed by measurements of vital capacity and blood gases.

Anticholinesterases such as neostigmine allow the level of acetylcholine at the motor end-plate to build up so that transmission will take place with improved muscle power. This is one of the principles of treatment. Mestinon (pyridostigmine) is another anticholinesterase commonly used because of its long action. Atropine may also need to be given to combat the muscarinic effects of the anticholinesterases (i.e. bradycardia, abdominal cramps from stimulation of the gut and excessive secretion of the glands of the mouth and lungs).

There are two situations where the myasthenic patient may require intensive care:

1 *Myasthenic crisis.* Here the myasthenic fails to respond to the normal dose of anticholinesterase because of a probable change in the sensitivity at the motor end-plate. IPPV will almost certainly be required initially through an endotracheal tube. Tracheostomy may well be necessary if the condition fails to resolve. Once control is obtained the patient can be taken off the ventilator and the effect on the tidal volume of 10 mg edrophonium (Tensilon) measured. An increase in tidal volume confirms the diagnosis. The test can also be made while the patient is still receiving IPPV by observing whether eye-opening and the strength of hand-grip are improved. It is often wise to ventilate the patient's lungs for a few days without anticholinesterases, and then start the drugs again possibly with the use of an IMV valve (page 80) or a triggering ventilator such as the Bird until confidence is regained. These patients may present a great problem and require long-term ventilation before muscle power returns.

2 *Cholinergic crisis.* Overdosage with anticholinesterase drugs may produce a depolarising block made worse with edrophonium. Excess salivation is often present in these cases and ventilation through a cuffed endotracheal tube will be required for several days without any anticholinesterase drugs. Treatment can then be re-established, but there is

often some difficulty in weaning from the ventilator. In both these complications, tube feeding will be necessary as swallowing will be affected. Chest infection is common and the appropriate antibiotic is required.

Thymectomy is often performed for myasthenia gravis and patients may require careful observation on the intensive care ward with emergency intubation instruments at hand. Patients who have had a sternal incision should be managed in the immediate postoperative period by elective IPPV.

Tetanus

Although rare, tetanus must always be considered when treating a convulsing patient. It is caused by a spore-bearing anaerobic bacterium *Clostridium tetani* producing a neurotoxin which travels up the perineural sheath of peripheral nerves. The toxin produces symptoms which vary from mild stiffness to major convulsions. The longer the time between infection and the onset of the first symptoms, the more favourable is the ultimate prognosis.

The causes of death in tetanus are from the following:

(a) hypoxia caused by the muscle spasm;
(b) chest infection due to under-ventilation and inhalation;
(c) pulmonary embolus;
(d) fulminating toxaemia;
(e) coincidental causes such as myocardial infarction.

Mild cases exhibiting local and minimal general stiffness without muscle spasms or opisthotonos may be treated by sedation alone. Diazepam may control these patients satisfactorily.

Moderate cases with generalised spasms, opisthotonos, and dysphagia will need tracheostomy in addition to sedation to allow suction and protect the airway. Chlorpromazine or diazepam may be used to control muscle spasms in these cases. Barbiturates are also useful to produce mental sedation. Intragastric tube feeding will be required.

Severe cases with multiple severe uncontrolled spasms associated with hypoxia will require tracheostomy and IPPV (see page 84). Muscle relaxants such as tubocurarine or pancuronium will be required to control spasms and to allow artificial ventilation. Adequate dosage at the slightest movement is required. Injections can be given intravenously or intramuscularly if possible. Diazepam or chlorpromazine given concurrently will sedate the patient and potentiate the muscle relaxants.

Patients with severe tetanus show excessive overactivity of the sympathetic nervous system. This instability is seen as marked fluctuations in heart rate and rhythm and blood pressure. Stimulation such as pharyngeal or tracheal suction, or turning, can provoke massive increases in heart rate and blood pressure. These effects can last for some considerable time after the stimulus has ceased. Profound hypotension may also occur. The sympathetic overactivity also produces an increased metabolic rate with profuse sweating, hyperpyrexia and extreme peripheral vaso-constriction. Beta-adrenergic receptor-blocking drugs such as propranolol may be required to attenuate the excessive sympathetic effects. Careful continuous monitoring of these patients is essential.

Surgical excision of any wound should be performed as early as possible under general anaesthesia. Human anti-tetanus immunoglobulin should be given to neutralise the circulating toxin. Large doses of antibiotics should be given to eliminate the source of toxin and to prevent complicating infections. Physiotherapy and nursing care will increase the chance of survival. Where possible, it is advisable to nurse these patients in a darkened quiet room, especially if the regime involves sedation alone.

Tube feeding should ensure adequate intake of fluid, calories, protein and vitamins. Accurate fluid balance charts should be kept.

At the end of 2 weeks, attempts should be made to wean the patient off the ventilator (see page 87) provided convulsions do not occur as the muscle relaxants wear off. In spite of treatment as outlined, the mortality rate may be as high as 25%.

Diagnosis of death

With modern intensive care techniques such as artificial ventilators and cardiac pacemakers, the diagnosis of death is increasingly difficult to establish. At one time, the cessation of heartbeat was all that was required and the failure of circulation rapidly resulted in cerebral death. Organ transplantation has made it vital for intensive care physicians to recognise *irreversible cerebral damage* before transplantable organs have been damaged by ischaemia. In addition, a decision may have to be made to discontinue artificial ventilation while the heart is still beating. These decisions involve ethical discussions but in the United Kingdom there is no legal definition of death and any action taken in any individual case in which respiration and beating heart are maintained solely by mechanical means is a matter for clinical judgement. The conclusion that respiration and a beating heart are being maintained solely by mechanical means and that brain death has occurred must be reached entirely independently of any transplant considerations. Nevertheless, once the diagnosis of death has been made the actual moment at which the mechanical supports are switched off may be influenced by the need to maintain organs other than the irreparably damaged brain in the best possible condition for eventual transplantation.

Various codes of practice have been devised to help in the diagnosis of brain death. The following is an abstract of the *Statement from the*

Conference of Medical Royal Colleges and their Faculties in the United Kingdom which was issued in 1976, with revision in 1981.

Conditions for considering diagnosis of brain death; all of the following should coexist:

1 the patient is deeply comatose;
2 the patient is being maintained on a lung ventilator because spontaneous respiration had previously become inadequate or had ceased altogether;
3 there should be no doubt that the patient's condition is due to irremediable structural brain damage. The diagnosis of a disorder which can lead to brain death should have been fully established.

It is essential to be sure that coma is not due to depressant drugs, bearing in mind that narcotics, hypnotics and tranquillisers may have prolonged durations of action. The effects can be potentiated in hypothermic patients. The benzodiazepine drugs (e.g. diazepam) are commonly used as anticonvulsants and to assist synchronisation with lung ventilators. These drugs act cumulatively and their effects persist in the body for days.

Other causes of coma should be excluded, such as primary hypothermia, metabolic and endocrine disturbances (e.g. profound abnormalities of the serum electrolytes, acid-base balance or blood glucose levels).

Muscle relaxants and similar drugs must have been excluded as a cause of respiratory inadequacy or failure.

It may take quite a long time to establish the diagnosis of brain death in patients who have suffered an indefinite period of cerebral hypoxia due to such causes as cardiac arrest, hypoxia, severe circulatory insufficiency, cerebral fat or air embolism. The diagnosis should be made by experienced clinicians; when the primary diagnosis is in doubt, a neurologist or neurosurgeon should be consulted. The tests which are used to confirm brain death should be carried out at a body temperature of not less than 35°C. A low-reading thermometer should be used. The diagnostic tests include those concerned with the brain-stem reflexes:

(a) fixed diameter pupils which do not respond to sharp changes in the intensity of light;

(b) absent corneal reflex;

(c) absent vestibulo-ocular reflexes—these reflexes are elicited during or after the slow instillation of 20 ml ice-cold water into each external auditory meatus, after clear access to the tympanic membrane has been established by visual inspection. (Local trauma on one or other side may contra-indicate this test);

(d) absent motor responses within the distribution of the cranial nerves after adequate stimulation of somatic areas;

(e) absent gag reflex, or reflex response to bronchial stimulation following stimulation by a suction catheter passed down the trachea;

(f) absent respiratory movements when the patient is disconnected from the mechanical ventilator for long enough to ensure that the $Paco_2$

rises above the threshold for stimulating respiration (i.e. above 50 mmHg or 6.7 kPa). If the patient is hypocapnic, carbon dioxide may be added to the inspired gas mixture to raise the arterial tension to the required level. Hypoxia during disconnection from the ventilator may be prevented by delivering 6 litres per minute of oxygen through a catheter into the trachea. In the absence of facilities for blood gas analysis, the ventilator can be supplied with pure oxygen for 10 minutes to pre-oxygenate the patient, then with 5 % carbon dioxide in oxygen for five minutes, and then disconnected for 10 minutes while delivering oxygen at 6 litres per minute by catheter into the trachea. This procedure establishes by diffusion oxygenation that hypoxia will not occur during the period of apnoea.

It is usual to repeat all the tests to be certain that there has been no observer error. The interval between the tests depends on the primary condition and the clinical cause of the disease.

Spinal cord function can persist for some time after the brain stem is irretrievably destroyed, and reflexes of spinal origin may persist or return after an initial absence in brain-dead patients. Electroencephalography (EEG) is not necessary for diagnosing brain death although it is valuable in the earlier stages of the care of patients. Figure 7.10 shows the normal relationships between electrical function, cerebral perfusion pressure and cerebral blood flow. Other investigations such as cerebral angiography or

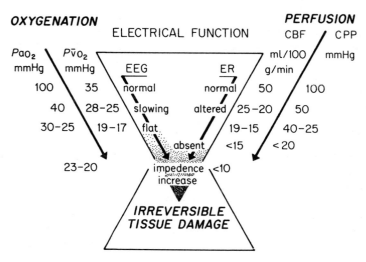

Fig. 7.10 Cerebral perfusion pressure (CPP) and cerebral blood flow (CBF) thresholds for changes in electroencephalogram (EEG) and evoked response (ER) activity. ER (i.e. a response to a specific stimulus) can be detected in the absence of a spontaneous EEG. However, neither measurement accurately predicts irreversible tissue damage. An increase in brain tissue impedance indicates sodium or potassium transport failure across the cell and may immediately precede cellular death

cerebral blood flow measurements are not required for diagnosis of brain death.

The decision to withdraw artifical support should be made after all the above criteria have been fulfilled. The following safeguards, which are normally observed by doctors concerned with such patients should be emphasised and form part of the guidelines to the profession, viz:

(a) The diagnosis of brain death should be made by two medical practitioners who have expertise in this field. One should be a consultant, the other being a consultant or senior registrar who should assure himself or herself that the preconditions have been met before testing is carried out. The length of time required before the preconditions can be satisfied varies according to the circumstances, and although occasionally it might be less than 24 hours it may extend to several days.

(b) The two doctors may carry out the tests separately or together. If the tests confirm brain death they should nevertheless be repeated. It is for the two doctors to decide how long the interval between tests should be but the time should be adequate for the reassurance of all those directly concerned.

(c) There may be circumstances in which it is impossible or inappropriate to carry out every one of the tests. The criteria published by the Conference of Medical Royal Colleges and their Faculties in the UK give recommended guidelines rather than rigid rules and it is for the doctors at the bedside to decide when the patient is dead.

8
Bleeding Problems

To understand and treat haemorrhagic conditions it is necessary to have a knowledge of the normal physiological haemostatic mechanisms. Bleeding may be mechanical from open vessels or non-mechanical when the bleeding occurs from cut tissue surfaces due to deficient physiological haemostatic mechanisms. Bleeding represents a defect in haemostasis, the process by which the body seals off leaks from the circulatory system. Haemostasis is a triple function depending on vascular integrity, platelet function and the coagulation mechanism.

Ligatures or sutures can control haemorrhage from major vessels, but only physiological haemostasis can check bleeding from the microvasculature. In the presence of deficient haemostatic mechanisms even the most careful mechanical haemostasis at operation will not prevent serious haemorrhage. With the development of modern surgical techniques, including cardiopulmonary bypass, massive blood replacement and organ transplantation, it has become apparent that some changes induced in the blood may become so extensive as to interfere with haemostasis.

Haemostasis

The requirements of haemostasis include a normal coagulation mechanism, intact vascular system and an adequate number of functioning platelets.

Platelets

The normal platelet count is 150 000 to 500 000 per mm^3. These small elements in the blood contain no nucleus and measure $2-4\ \mu m$ in diameter. They are formed in the haemopoietic marrow, the parent cell being the megakaryocyte. Platelets are very adhesive and as soon as an endothelial deficiency occurs in a blood vessel they adhere to the denuded area at the site of the injury to seal it off. Vasoactive substances are released from the platelets, initiating vasospasm and fibrin deposition. The platelet aggregate fuses into a solid plug; this sequence of platelet activity is known as the *primary haemostatic response*. This is the manner by which bleeding from the capillaries and small arterioles of a surgical incision is initially controlled.

Platelets are also responsible for maintaining capillary wall impermeability and they play a part in clot retraction, which has an important haemostatic action.

The coagulation mechanism

The outward simplicity of blood coagulation covers a remarkable series of events. The central process in clotting is the activation of prothrombin to thrombin. Thrombin is the enzyme which initiates platelet aggregation and induces fibrin formation. Fibrin forms the major scaffolding structure of a blood clot.

The clotting mechanism is essentially a sequence of enzyme reactions that can be compared to a line of falling dominoes; if one falls it will knock over the next and so on until all the line has fallen over. The concentration of the enzymes increases as the clotting sequence proceeds, the earlier steps taking more time than the latter ones. The clotting factors are plasma proteins, many of them present in only trace amounts. It is usual to recognise that blood clotting can occur in two ways and the clotting mechanism is subdivided into two systems (see Fig. 8.1):

1 The intrinsic system. All the components of this system are present in the plasma and clotting will occur when blood comes into contact with wettable surfaces, e.g. glass, vascular prostheses, heart-lung or kidney machines as well as severe atheroscleroses. The sequence is easy to remember as the clotting factors are involved in descending order, except that factor X is displaced. The sequence is XII, XI, IX, VIII, X, II, and I.

2 The extrinsic system. This is initiated by tissue damage when there is release of tissue factor III into the blood, e.g. trauma, burns and operations. This factor, with the help of factor VII, activates factor X *and thus the terminal part of the two clotting systems is a common pathway.*

There are many synonyms for the different clotting factors but for clarity the internationally designated Roman numerals should be used (Table 8.1).

Plasminogen

This is a protein which is found in plasma. It is a precursor of plasmin, a proteolytic enzyme, which will break down fibrin and some other clotting factors (fibrinolysis). This indicates that there is an opposing fibrinolytic enzyme system which is a defence mechanism against intravascular coagulation.

Defects in haemostasis

1 Vascular defects

The majority of causes of bleeding from inborn vascular defects rarely cause haemorrhage significant enough to necessitate intensive care.

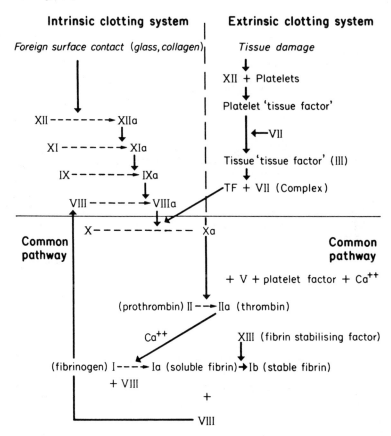

Fig. 8.1 The domino or cascade representation of clotting reactions. The suffix 'a' denotes the active enzyme form of each factor. Factor X is activated by the intrinsic system and by the extrinsic system. Thrombin also acts on the platelets to release phospholipid and on factor VIII first to stabilise it then to destroy it

However, in the postoperative patient who is bleeding significantly it is essential to distinguish between surgical haemorrhage from damaged blood vessels, which require surgical ligation, and bleeding due to a haemostatic defect, which requires specific therapy to correct the deficit. Inborn vascular defects which may be responsible for severe haemorrhage are met with when there is fragility and hyperelasticity of connective tissues, such as Ehlers-Danlos syndrome, Cushing's syndrome and Marfan's syndrome.

2 Platelet defects

The platelet abnormality may affect the vascular endothelium as well as the coagulation of blood and accounts for a number of clinical problems.

Table 8.1 Clotting factors

Factor:	
I	fibrinogen
II	prothrombin
III	thromboplastin (tissue factor)
IV	ionic calcium (Ca^{++})
V	labile factor
No factor VI	
VII	proconvertin (stable factor)
VIII	antihaemophilic globulin (AHG)
IX	Christmas factor
X	Stuart factor
XI	plasma thromboplastin antecedent (PTA)
XII	Hageman (or contact) factor
XIII	Fibrin stabilising factor (FSF)

NB All the clotting factors except IV and VIII are formed in the liver

The platelets may be too few (thrombocytopenia) or the number may be normal but of defective function (thrombopathy), e.g. von Willebrand's disease. Thrombocytopenia is by far the commonest of the two and bleeding may develop when the count falls below 60 000 per mm³. Bleeding may occur anywhere but particularly affects the subcutaneous tissues, intestines, urinary tract and central nervous system (CNS).

Investigation of thrombocytopenic patients should include peripheral blood smears for leukaemia and lupus erythematosus, biopsy of any enlarged lymph nodes to exclude sarcoidosis or lymphoma, and a bone marrow aspiration to determine the functional state of the mega-karyocytes and to rule out malignant bone marrow invasion. Depression of bone marrow function may follow radiation or drug therapy.

Drugs known to be capable of inducing thrombocytopenia include:

Sedatives—meprobamate, phenobarbitone;

Antibiotics—oxytetracycline, chloramphenicol, streptomycin, para-aminosalicylic acid, most of the antibacterial sulphonamides and some of the sulphonamide derivatives, e.g. chlorothiazide, acetazolamide (Diamox), chlorpropamide (Diabinese);

Other agents—quinidine, quinine, digoxin, oestrogens, thiourea, gold, mercurials, bismuth and arsenicals.

It is thought that in the majority of cases drug-induced thrombocytopenia is due to sensitivity reactions. The usual manifestations are chills, fever, lethargy, pruritis, gum-bleeding, epistaxis, petechiae, shock and finally severe haemorrhage most usually into the CNS and renal or gastro-intestinal tracts. In burns, thrombocytopenia may develop within several hours of the injury. Treatment of bleeding due to platelet deficiency is to identify and treat the causative factor if possible. If transfusion is necessary fresh blood obtained in siliconised or plastic containers, which conserve the platelets or platelet concentrates, should be used.

3 Coagulation disorders

Most clotting disorders are acquired. One acquired cause of bleeding that may be seen in patients receiving intensive care is due to intestinal sterilisation. The intestinal flora are a major source of vitamin K in man. Patients who have their gastrointestinal tracts sterilised by large doses of antibiotics lose this source of vitamin K which is essential for the formation of prothrombin by the liver.

Massive transfusion. Factors V and VIII and platelets are deficient in stored blood. The factors decrease after 21 days of storage to 20–50 % and so are largely a primary cause of bleeding. However, the haemostatic effectiveness of platelets rapidly decays over 48–72 hours. Platelet concentrations or fresh whole blood, both of which contain viable platelets, will correct bleeding due to dilutional thrombocytopenia.

Haemophilia. Classical haemophilia due to deficiency in factor VIII (antihaemophilic globulin or AHG) is the most important, most common and most serious bleeding disorder. Approximately 1 in 10 000 people is affected by the disease, less than one-half being seriously affected. As factor VIII is concerned only in the intrinsic clotting pathway, a prolonged kaolin-cephalin time (see page 168) but a normal prothrombin time is found. Since the extrinsic pathway is not affected, the blood clots readily on contact with tissues and massive clots can form. However, there is no significant haemostatic effect as there is no clotting in direct relationship to the vessel wall defect.

As in most physiological processes, there is a large safety margin with normal AHG levels. A haemophilic patient rarely bleeds unless the AHG level falls below 5 % of normal. In severe cases when the level of AHG is consistently around 1 % few survive beyond childhood, death usually resulting from CNS or gastrointestinal haemorrhage. In the moderate (1– 5 %) or mild (5–25 %) groups, the major bleeding problems usually arise after even minor trauma or operation. These cases need specialist management by a haematologist.

The disease is genetically sex-linked, the female being the carrier and only males being frank haemophiliacs. Briefly, the specific care necessary in these patients, in addition to the problem of hypovolaemia due to bleeding, is to maintain a satisfactory AHG level in the blood by transfusion of factor VIII preparation. The factor VIII level should be maintained ideally at 40–80 % in the first few days after trauma or surgery or if bleeding is occurring. This level is not easily attained and management is difficult with recurrent bleeding still being a significant problem. A level of 30 % is the minimum necessary to secure haemostasis after major operations. The level of factor VIII in these patients may fluctuate and is related to the rate of its utilisation. This is affected by the metabolic rate which in turn in related to the temperature, and stress conditions of operation or trauma. The severity of the condition must be checked regularly by factor VIII assays or kaolin-cephalin times (p. 168).

An identical clinical picture is found in patients suffering from factor IX deficiency (Christmas disease). Factor IX concentrates prepared from human plasma are available for treatment.

4   Disseminated Intravascular Coagulation (DIC)

This syndrome has recently stimulated considerable interest when it was realised that it is the most frequently acquired haemostatic defect. It is also referred to as consumption coagulopathy or acute defibrination syndrome. DIC is characterised by the development of a low or absent fibrinogen level in the blood and thrombocytopenia. If this occurs in relationship to an operation severe bleeding can ensue. The low fibrinogen level rarely results from defective fibrinogen production. It is virtually always due to rapid utilisation of the fibrinogen by intravascular coagulation or its destruction by fibrinolysis. These two processes usually occur simultaneously.

DIC results from activation of one or several of the following processes:

(a) activation of the Hageman (contact) factor and the intrinsic coagulation system because of the damage to endothelial cells;

(b) activation of the extrinsic coagulation system because of injury to tissues;

(c) release of phospholipids (which cause coagulation) because of injury to platelets or red blood cells.

The aggregates formed by platelet damage are filtered off in the microvascular bed where they stimulate local coagulation with fibrin formation. If the process continues there is progressive tissue ischaemia as the vascular bed becomes increasingly obstructed. The response to this obstruction is a rapid local fibrinolysis which is aimed at maintaining the patency of the microcirculation. The re-opening of these vascular channels is associated with the release of excessive amounts of soluble fibrin degradation ('split') products into the systemic circulation. Accumulation of these products causes serious derangements of coagulation and haemostatic function, with the clinical manifestations of a general haemorrhagic state (Fig. 8.2). This is due to loss of platelets and consumption of factors V and VII.

DIC is a selected group of syndromes associated with excessive or pathological forms of fibrinogen derivatives which are usually due to proteolysis. Patients usually present with a bleeding problem somewhere in the body. In a minority of cases (2 %) there is clinical thrombosis. The

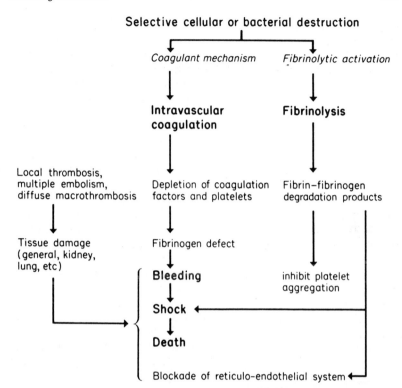

Fig. 8.2 Processes involved in Disseminated Intravascular Coagulation (DIC)

obstetric causes may include abruptio placenta, dead fetus syndrome, amniotic fluid embolism, eclampsia, miscarriage or abortion, especially septic. The surgical causes include trauma, pneumonectomy, graft surgery and transplantation. DIC may also occur in carcinomatosis and leukaemia. It is not often realised that the prime cause of death following an incompatible blood transfusion is because of DIC. The process predominantly affects the kidneys, lungs and liver. Clinically, there is progressive acidosis, oedema, haemorrhage and progressive lung, liver and renal failure (hepato-renal syndrome). Intravascular haemolysis also occurs. Intestinal manifestations are haemorrhagic gastritis and endocolitis. Infections, especially septicaemia, may also give rise to DIC.

The effects of DIC are related to the organs which are involved: cardiac involvement may be shown by dysrhythmias, infarction or even arrest; lung involvement is shown by hypoxia, haemoptysis or the adult form of respiratory distress syndrome ('shock lung', 'DIC lung', page 94).

Treatment. DIC is a paradox in that bleeding and thrombosis are occurring simultaneously and are further complicated by another paradox in that one of the recommended forms of treatment of the haemorrhage is the administration of the anticoagulant heparin. DIC is never a primary disease state, nor will it develop in every patient who suffers from one of the recognised causes.

Central nervous system disorder may be shown by coma with focal signs, bleeding or embolic phenomena; kidney involvement results in oliguria or anuria.

There is no one pathognomonic laboratory test to diagnose DIC. The laboratory tests which are going to be useful are the quick ones because there is no point in getting results back a day or two afterwards. The quick tests include assay of platelets, fibrinogen, thrombin time, prothrombin time, activated partial thromboplastin time, fibrin degradation products, factors V and VIII. Blood gas and acid-base analysis are used to monitor the progress of the illness. A fall in platelet count, however, is *not* necessarily a diagnostic feature, but the same could really be said about any of these tests.

Most attention has been given to treatment with heparin, antibiotics, corticosteroids and transfusion of blood products. It is difficult to establish whether any of these treatments really does help avert the progress of the syndrome. Heparin was thought to be a useful treatment. Indeed laboratory tests may return to normal during heparin treatment, but patients may still die. If heparin does help, then it needs to be given immediately. If epsilon aminocaproic acid (Epsikapron, EACA), tranexamic acid (Cyclokapron) or similar agents are used to inhibit fibrinolysis, a fatal outcome due to massive intravascular thrombosis is likely unless heparin therapy has been given first.

Claims have been made for the efficacy of streptokinase in patients with severe abnormal haematological tests. The mainstay of treatment is to treat infection and the underlying condition where possible, to maintain blood volume and to replace missing blood factors.

Management of bleeding problems

Any suspicion of a bleeding tendency in a patient's history should be investigated before operation. A single test to detect abnormalities of the haemostatic mechanism is not available. There are, however, only two basic tests which are widely used:

1 *The kaolin-cephalin time*, which estimates the activity of the intrinsic clotting system. Prolongation of this clotting time is almost always due to deficiency of factor VIII or IX (haemophilia or Christmas disease respectively).

2 *The prothrombin time*, which estimates the activity of the extrinsic system. This test is chiefly sensitive to deficiency of factors V, VII and X.

In all clotting tests the clotting time is compared on each occasion with a normal plasma since there are always small differences in the activities of the reagents that are used. Further tests are available to identify accurately practically every conceivable abnormality. A defect can almost always be corrected once its nature has been established.

Once bleeding has developed, treatment by blood transfusion must usually be resorted to before these tests can be started or completed. In these circumstances citrated blood should be routinely collected before transfusion is commenced to enable subsequent accurate testing. A specimen should be collected by a single, clean venepuncture using a plastic syringe without the use of a tourniquet. The blood container should be immediately cooled at $4°C$ and transferred to the haematological laboratory. The immediate treatment of serious bleeding is the replacement of blood loss to maintain an adequate blood volume. This may involve massive transfusion of bank blood, often aggravating the bleeding due to exhaustion of factors V and VIII which are virtually absent in bank blood. This is a very common complication of blood replacement for cases of severe haemorrhage and every attempt should be made to obtain as much fresh blood as possible. If fresh blood is not available, the transfused bank blood will need supplementing by units of fresh frozen plasma which contain the thermolabile factors V and VIII not present in bank blood. Close collaboration with the haematological laboratory is vital.

Cardiopulmonary bypass

Blood is traumatised as it passes through the heart-lung machine, with denaturation of plasma proteins and destruction of platelets and erythrocytes. There is a decline in fibrinogen and prothrombin levels and these changes increase as the bypass time increases. These patients are at special risk from postoperative haemorrhage and any abnormally serious bleeding can rapidly exhaust clotting factors to such an extent that the resulting complex clotting derangement cannot be corrected and a lethal haemorrhagic vicious circle develops. In addition, these cases are particularly prone to suffer from fibrinolysis and intravascular coagulation problems. During and after a cardiopulmonary bypass with a 'non-blood prime' in the heart-lung machine, the concentration of coagulation factors is low due to the dilutional effect.

Other conditions predispose the patient to postoperative haemorrhagic states of a similar nature. These include extensive resections for cancer, especially prostate, lung, breast and pancreas, fibrinolysis being the commonest clotting abnormality.

Management of severe haemorrhage

If postoperative or post-traumatic bleeding occurs it must be ensured that a major vessel defect is not the cause. Postoperative haemorrhage from wounds or chest tubes probably results more often from the latter than from a deranged clotting mechanism. In emergency situations it is often difficult to define the exact cause of the bleeding. An abnormal bleeding or clotting time and the presence of petechiae or ecchymoses indicate an abnormal haemostatic mechanism, but the absence of these does not absolve the mechanism. Proper testing is required to exclude an abnormal haemostatic mechanism and this should be done in close collaboration with the haematological department. This stresses the importance of accurate investigation of all bleeding problems and in outline the investigations fall into three main groups:

1 Platelet tests.
2 Clotting tests.
3 Tests for fibrinolysis and hypercoagulation.

In the emergency conditions of severe haemorrhage it is important to maintain the blood volume and at the same time not allow aggravation of the condition by clotting factor exhaustion. This is why fresh blood, fresh frozen plasma or special plasma fractions should be used. Cryoprecipitate is a protein selectively rich in fibrinogen and factor VIII.

9
Nutritional Support

The object of nutritional support is to provide the basic food materials for body homeostasis when normal alimentation is not possible. This is a common necessity in the ICU. Daily energy requirements are shown in Table 9.1.

Virtually all patients requiring intensive care are in a catabolic state—that is they are breaking down body tissues due to an activated metabolic response to injury. This response is related to a dual hormonal response:

1 The initial acute phase is mediated through the sympathetic system. Catecholamines are released from the adrenal medulla and sympathetic nerve endings, causing inhibition of insulin secretion and stimulation of glucagon secretion. In addition, there is an increased adrenocorticotropic hormone (ACTH) release from the pituitary which stimulates release of the adrenocortical hormones. This all results in protein breakdown, new formation of glucose and fat oxidation. This acute phase usually lasts for one to five days but can be much longer and the duration is related to the severity of the onslaught on the patient.

2 An anabolic adaptive phase follows, when the crisis is over. Insulin levels are lower, blood glucose falls and the concentrations of catecholamines and glucorticoids in the plasma return to normal. This 'rebuilding' phase is associated with increasing utilisation of body fat.

Table 9.1 Approximate 24 hour energy requirements for 70 kg adult

	Starving but non-catabolic state	Catabolic state	Hypercatabolic state
Nitrogen g*	7.5	14	25
kcal (total) including protein	2000	3000	4000
Non-protein kcal/g nitrogen	250	200	135

NB   1 kcal = 4.1868 kilojoules, kj; 1000 kcal = 4.1868 megajoules, MJ;
     1 MJ = 238.8 kcal

* Nitrogen = protein in g ÷ 6.25

This metabolic response to trauma causes diminution of muscle mass and plasma proteins with impaired immune response to infection and delay in wound healing. Even elective surgical procedures can transform mild categories of malnutrition into significant states which adversely affect ultimate recovery. Fifty per cent of patients who have had major operations more than seven days earlier show evidence of protein-calorie malnutrition.

The nutritional status of a patient can be assessed by simple tests among which are:

(a) weight loss greater than 10 % of ideal weight;
(b) mid-triceps arm circumference less than 23 cm in males and 22 cm in women;
(c) mid-triceps skinfold thickness less than 10 mm in men and 13 mm in women;
(d) lymphocyte count less than 1500/mm^3;
(e) serum albumin less than 35 g/l.

It has been demonstrated that the planned administration of protein covered by a large calorific intake can markedly reduce the breakdown of body muscle. The amount of urinary 'leakage' of an infused load of amino acids is no higher than 15 %, supporting the view that infused amino acids can be utilised by the body.

In the previously healthy adult a period of two to five days starvation is often well tolerated, energy requirements being supplied from the patient's body fat and protein. However, this, in conjunction with a period of catabolic stress, is a much more serious matter. Postoperative morbidity and length of stay in hospital are reduced in patients receiving intensive and immediate postoperative feeding. In the critically ill patient these considerations are even more important.

Energy reserves are relatively smaller in the child and one day's starvation is the maximum that should be allowed, although in the newborn there is a natural reserve of 48 hours labile fat and protein.

The percentage of the body's labile protein is small and when this supply has been used fixed tissue protein such as muscle is then catabolised to provide essential amino acids. Only approximately 20 % of calories produced are derived from fat and 35 % results from the breakdown of fat-free sources. The increased metabolism is aggravated further by fever, infection, anaemia, acidosis and hypoxia. When such conditions prevail the loss of body tissue becomes a major factor. Survival is exceptional when more than 30 % of the ideal body weight has been lost. Inadequate protein-calorie intake is a consistent problem in all patients under intensive care when oral feeding is not possible.

Alimentary dysfunction may follow any operation. It is most common after abdominal surgery, and in any form of shock gastrointestinal function may cease. In this condition it is important to establish gastric drainage by passing a stomach tube. This ensures that gastric dilatation does not occur with the attendant risk of sudden torrential regurgitation and respiratory inhalation. In addition, gastric aspiration measurements allow assessment of fluid and electrolyte loss into the bowel and when gastrointestinal function returns the gastric aspirate will reduce to negligible levels indicating that enteral feeding can be commenced.

When gastric drainage is required, a radio-opaque tipped nasogastric tube should be passed via the nose and an X-ray taken to confirm its correct position in the stomach. It is usual to aspirate the stomach every hour or so and in the intervening periods the tube should be left open to free drainage.

Enteral feeding

If gastrointestinal function is intact but swallowing impossible, the insertion of a nasogastric or nasoduodenal feeding tube with subsequent feeding through the tube is the best method of nutritional support (enteral feeding). Once it has been established that gastrointestinal absorption is satisfactory, the relatively uncomfortable large-bore tube can be replaced by a fine bore (1 mm) feeding tube and continuous gravity or roller pump feeding commenced through this tube. This is advantageous because it saves nursing time, is much more comfortable for the patient and these fine bore tubes do not appear to cause oesophageal erosions, ulcers or strictures. Also, continuous slow-rate feeding is less associated with troublesome diarrhoea.

In patients where the oesophagus is not intact a feeding gastrostomy or jejunostomy is indicated.

When feeding is commenced a starter regimen is advisable. At first, water is given at the rate of up to 30 ml/h. At this stage it is usual to aspirate the tube gently before insertion of the next feed. Within a few hours it is obvious if the fluid offered is being absorbed. If it is, the fluid volume should be progressively increased and at the same time the fluid should be augmented to half-strength feeds. The mixture is then changed to full-strength feed.

A balanced low residue diet comprising carbohydrates, proteins, water, electrolytes, trace elements and vitamins should be established, affording the order of 3000 kcal/day in a 2–3 litre volume. The feed should be made up by the dietitian ensuring sterility and suitable consistency for tube feeding. Regular bacterial culture checks should be made of feed samples as it is surprising how often a pathogen such as *Pyocyaneus* is isolated. Infected feeds can be a troublesome cause of bowel irritation and inflammation.

Proprietary enteral feed preparations. Various proprietary feed preparations are available and have the advantage of guaranteed sterility.

There are two distinct commercial preparations:

1 whole protein preparations;
2 elemental feeds where free amino acids represent the nitrogen source.

The whole protein preparations are preferable (and cheaper) except in patients with pancreatic deficiency or with reduced bowel absorption surface, such as short bowel syndrome.

Vitamin, electrolyte and trace element contents of the listed products (Table 9.2) are adequate but may have to be supplemented in patients who are losing large volumes of fluid.

The management of enteral feeding must be based on the clinical details of the patient. Assessment of nitrogen balance from blood and urine specimens should be performed twice-weekly and regular weighing of the patient by bed balance technique and nutritional assessment should also be regularly performed. The catabolic patient requires less calories per gram of nitrogen than the non-catabolic patient. If the calorie-nitrogen balance of feed requires modification in proprietary preparations, additional energy can be added by means of calorie feeds such as Caloreen.

Complications

Diarrhoea is the most common complication of enteral feeding. It is most commonly associated with too rapid an introduction of the feed, especially that of high osmolality; about 1 kcal/ml of solution is the most that can be tolerated. Other causes are infected feeds, lactose intolerance and antibiotic therapy. If diarrhoea persists despite exclusion of possible causes, addition of codeine phosphate will usually control the tendency.

It is common for the catabolic patient to show glucose intolerance due to impaired intrinsic insulin production and insulin 'resistance'. Regular blood glucose measurements should be performed and insulin given if necessary to maintain acceptable blood sugar levels.

Total parenteral nutrition (TPN)

When normal alimentary function is not present, parenteral nutrition is necessary. The introduction of TPN carries with it the need for increased awareness of complications including hyperosmolar states and rebound hypoglycaemia. It is essential to ensure that a planned regime is employed in order to achieve the best results. One of the most serious biochemical complications of intravenous feeding with essential amino acids and glucose alone is hypophosphataemia. Protein must be supplied with appropriate amounts of calories so that resynthesis of body protein can occur without a breakdown of the administered amino acid for the

Table 9.2 Enteral preparations

Product	Non-nitrogen calories to nitrogen ratio	Lactose content	Osmolarity mOsmol/litre	Energy kcal/undiluted product
Clinifeed Iso (Roussel)	200:1	Yes	270 (undil.)	375 kcal/375 ml
Clinifeed 400 (Roussel)	142:1	Yes	346 (undil.) 255 (dil. to 500 ml)	400 kcal/375 ml
Clinifeed *neutral/coffee* (Roussel)	145:1	No	365 (undil.)	375 kcal/375 ml
Protein-rich Clinifeed (Roussel)	79:1	Yes	562 (undil.) 399 (dil. to 500 ml)	500 kcal/375 ml
Clinifeed Select *beef and carrot* (Roussel)	115:1	No	532 (undil.) 387 (dil. to 500 ml)	500 kcal/375 ml
Ensure (Abbott Labs)	148:1	No	380 (undil.) 190 (dil. 1:1 with water)	240 kcal/235 ml
Ensure Plus (Abbott Labs)	140:1	No	460 (undil.) 230 (dil. 1:1 with water)	340 kcal/235 ml
Isocal (Mead Johnson)	167:1	No	250 (undil.)	251 kcal/237 ml
Nutrauxil (KabiVitrum)	141:1	Trace	300 (undil.)	500 kcal/500 ml

All the above products are gluten-free and contain nitrogen from a whole protein source.

NB This data is correct at time of going to print but up-to-date manufacturer's information must be consulted before using any of the above feeds.
Full product information will also ensure that the feed meets requirements in other respects e.g. electrolytes, vitamins and minerals.

provision of energy requirements. A minimum of 2000 kcal (30–50 kcal/kg of body weight) are required per day. This should include 60 g or more of protein and at least 30 % of the calories should come from carbohydrates. Two basic preparations are required:

1 solutions containing nitrogen;
2 readily available calorie solution.

The nitrogen solution of amino acids is available as Aminoplex 12, Trophysan or Vamin. If potassium is supplied together with the amino acid there is greater utilisation of the nitrogen. The calorie solutions available include glucose, fructose, dextrose and sorbitol. Although fructose has been widely used as a substitute for glucose, its exact role in intravenous feeding remains controversial. Sorbitol is a sugar alcohol which has been widely used but it is converted to fructose and glucose, and apart from a higher calorie yield it provides no metabolic advantage over glucose. The advantages claimed for fructose and sorbitol are that they do not require the action of insulin for their metabolism and their use in hypertonic solutions is not usually associated with hyperglycaemia. The disadvantage of all carbohydrate solutions is the high concentration which has to be used in order to supply sufficient calories without an excess of water. They are all acidic with a pH 3.5–4.5 and cause local vein irritation and thrombosis.

The complications of the use of alcohol in TPN are now so many that its use should be discouraged.

Fat emulsions

Fat emulsions prepared from soya bean oil (e.g. Intralipid, KabiVitrum) are free from serious side effects and are safe to use. They provide a means of combining a high calorie infusion with a limited fluid volume as well as having a physiological pH, and are best reserved for use when high osmolar loads are unwise. Intravenously administered fat emulsion is rapidly metabolised, but several days of adaptation are required to obtain maximal utilisation.

Administration. These preparations should be administered through a central venous catheter dedicated to parenteral feeding. Peripheral vein cannulae can be used but the site must be changed frequently to prevent thrombophlebitis. The balance of nitrogen to calories is important and should be of the order of 0.2 g of amino acid nitrogen and 35–50 kcal/kg body weight/day. In order to achieve this it is usually necessary to use fat emulsions. Full parenteral nutrition can be maintained by 1–15 litres of 20% fat emulsion together with 1 litre of 10% amino acid hydrolysate per day. Additional fluids can be given to provide a daily total of 3–3.5 litres by the addition of 0.5–1.0 litres of 20% fructose. Sodium is included in the amino acid solution. If a low salt input is necessary, pure synthetic amino acid preparations are available, e.g. Trophysan, Aminoplex 12 or Vamin, which have very low salt content. Vamin or Aminoplex 12 are preferred to Trophysan as the amino acids are all in the pure laevo form and are therefore available for metabolic building.

Preparations available for parenteral infusion. These include:

(i) *Aminoplex 12 (Geistlich)*, a solution of synthetic laevo-form amino acids in 500 ml or 1000 ml glass bottles containing 12.4 g nitrogen/l,

30 mmol potassium/l, 35 mmol sodium/l. The energy content is 325 kcal/l and the pH of the solution is 7.4.

(ii) *Vamin glucose (KabiVitrum)* in bottles of 500 ml contains 650 kcal/l, 9.4 g nitrogen/l, 50 mmol sodium/l and 20 mmol potassium/l. The pH of the solution is 5.2. Vamin 'N is the same but contains only 250 kcal/l.

(iii) *Aminoplex 5 (Geistlich)* solution provides a full complement of calories and laevo amino acids together with balanced electrolytes suitable for repeated-sequence parenteral feeding in non-catabolic patients. It is supplied in 1000 ml glass bottles, containing 5 g nitrogen/l and 1000 kcal/l in the form of sorbitol and ethanol, sodium 35 mmol/l and potassium 15 mmol/l.

(iv) *Intralipid 20%* in bottles of 500 ml provides 2000 kcal/l but no electrolytes at pH 7.

(v) *Intralipid 10%* in bottles of 500 ml provides 1100 kcal/l at pH 7.

A typical adult regimen is outlined in Table 9.3. It is helpful to administer the fat emulsion and amino acid solution simultaneously because this is associated with better assimilation; a Y-connection can be used.

It is important, when maintaining patients by parenteral nutrition, to collect and analyse all excreta for electrolyte and nitrogen content. By this means the daily loss of electrolytes can be measured and suitably replaced. Potassium is of particular importance as it is essential that an adequate supply is available for protein resynthesis. In long-term parenteral nutrition other minerals such as calcium and magnesium should be added; full vitamin supplements are also necessary. At least fourteen trace elements are known to be required for the normal growth and develop-

Table 9.3 A typical adult regimen for parenteral infusion

Solution	kcal	Time
500 ml 20% fructose + 15 mmol KCl	400	4 hours
500 ml 10% Aminoplex 12 + 15 mmol KCl ⎫ 500 ml 20% Intralipid + 10 mg heparin ⎬	1000	6 hours
500 ml 20% fructose + 15 mmol KCl	400	4 hours
500 ml 10% Aminoplex 12 + 15 mmol KCl ⎫ 500 ml 20% Intralipid + 10 mg heparin ⎬	1000	6 hours
500 ml 20% fructose + 15 mmol KCl	400	4 hours
3.5 litres	3200 (12.5 g nitrogen)	24 hours

ment of one or more animal species. Many of these elements have only recently been considered as essential and all play a part in the regulation of biochemical pathways. It has been customary to consider only seven of these elements (cobalt, copper, iron, iodine, fluorine, manganese and zinc) as important in human nutrition.

General considerations

Patients in stress states are often strongly catabolic and it may be impossible to convert them to a positive calorific balance. The administration of 10–14 g of nitrogen per day, however, represents a sparing of lean body mass which would otherwise be catabolised and is of considerable benefit to the patient. In patients with severe illnesses following major trauma or operation the prevention of simple starvation by parenteral feeding may be the deciding factor in ultimate survival. There is an increased turnover of albumin in these cases and it is difficult to maintain normal concentration of the albumin by parenteral nutrition. Intermittent infusions of 100–150 g of albumin may be necessary to maintain protein levels in the serum at a level of not less than 30 g/l.

Complications

During the administration of fat emulsion the serum becomes turbid. This usually clears within three to four hours of completion of the infusion. The turbid serum can produce technical difficulties during routine biochemical or haematological tests and any blood samples should be taken during clear fluid infusion periods. Fat emulsions are contraindicated in septic patients and in hepatocellular jaundice.

Thrombophlebitis is not uncommon and is minimised by utilisation of a central venous catheter and adding 1000 units (10 mg) of heparin to each 500 ml of fat suspension. In addition, during the administration of fat emulsion hypercoagulability of blood can occur and these changes are reversed by the administration of the small quantities of heparin. The addition of heparin has the further advantage of increasing the rate of clearance of fat emulsion from the serum as it increases the activity of the enzyme lipoprotein lipase in the serum.

Addition of drugs to solutions used in parenteral nutrition

The success of intravenous feeding depends on safe access to the circulation over a considerable period of time. Thrombophlebitis and septicaemia are serious problems. Clearly, poor technique is the cause of infection and thrombophlebitis, and only careful attention to detail of catheter insertion and maintenance of the infusion can combat the problem. It must be emphasised that parenteral nutrition catheters should never be used for blood sampling, blood transfusion or intermittent intravenous therapy. No substances other than heparin should be added to Intralipid because of the danger of flocculation. Aminosol may be mixed with Intralipid by way of the Y-tube as already described.

The addition of any drugs or electrolytes to Aminosol should be by a rigidly aseptic technique as the amino acid solution is a good broth for bacterial growth. Some amino acid solutions will support the growth of *Candida albicans* even at body temperature. Aminosol solutions have a pH of about 5, which may cause precipitation of poorly-soluble weak acids, such as penicillins and fusidic acid (Fucidin), and these should not be added.

Bacterial contamination of nutrient solutions is a serious problem and can occur when adding electrolytes or trace elements to bottles of amino acids. The addition of electrolytes or the mixing of nutrients must be made in a pharmacy by a faultless technique.

Patients may develop septicaemia without any local signs of thrombo-phlebitis. A swinging temperature and positive blood cultures suggest septic emboli from an infected thrombus around the tip of the catheter. If no other obvious causes for the infection are found, the catheter should be removed, the clot cultured and appropriate antibiotics given.

The junction between the catheter and the skin should be kept bacteriologically clear by repeated cleaning or use of occlusive antiseptic dressings. Successful long-term parenteral nutrition has been aided by the use of soft silicone rubber catheters introduced into the superior vena cava via a peripheral vein. The surgical procedure involves placement of the catheter in a long subcutaneous tunnel before it enters the vein. A Dacron cuff on the catheter becomes fixed in the subcutaneous tissues by fibrous tissue and forms a barrier to the entry of organisms.

10

Nursing Care and Procedures

The respiratory system

Oral or nasal tracheal intubation

This procedure should be undertaken only by a nurse who has received special training and is skilled in the procedure.

A record should always be kept of the size of the endotracheal tube used, and one of the same type and size with the equipment necessary for emergency reintubation and hand ventilation should be kept by the patient's bedside at all times. If a rubber tube has been used in an emergency procedure it is preferable to change it to a plastic type with a low-pressure soft cuff as soon as possible. If endotracheal intubation is to be maintained for prolonged periods the tube is usually changed at regular intervals by the anaesthetist and the larynx examined under direct vision at the same time.

A nurse's duties in connection with endotracheal tubes must be meticulously performed, the patient's life depending on instant recognition of any faults. Signs of complications arising in relation to the endotracheal and breathing tubes and their connections include changes in the following:

(a) the patient's colour, pulse and blood pressure;
(b) his level of consciousness and appearance of agitation or anxiety;
(c) tidal volume or minute volume recordings;
(d) respiratory rate, effort and movement;
(e) pressures within the breathing circuit;
(f) temperature and sweating;
(g) amount, colour and appearance of aspirate.

The cuff of the tube is best inflated with a 10 ml syringe (Fig. 10.1). The volume used should just exclude air-escape around the tube in a patient who is unable to cough or whose lungs are being ventilated. Under-inflation of the cuff will result in under-ventilation if the patient is on intermittent positive pressure ventilation (IPPV) and over-inflation will produce an excessive pressure on the tracheal mucous membrane, resulting in tracheal damage with the risk of ulceration, haemorrhage or tracheal stricture. When the cuff is correctly inflated there will be no noise of escaping air—this, when present, usually produces a clearly audible 'gurgle'. Small leaks from the cuff tubing may occur and if frequent cuff inflation is required, or if at any time a volume in excess of 10 ml is needed to gain a seal, the anaesthetist must be called. In such circumstances the endotracheal tube may require changing because it is defective or too

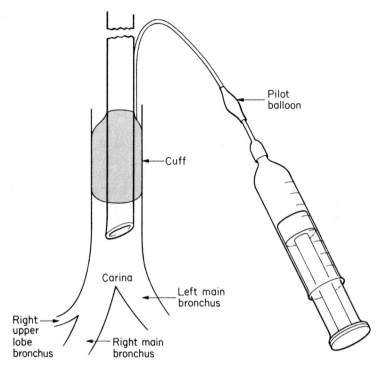

Fig. 10.1 A correctly placed endotracheal tube with the cuff inflated

small, or it may indicate that serious pathological changes are occurring in the tracheal wall. If intubation is required for longer than seven to ten days a tracheostomy or cricothyroidotomy is often performed and the same caution is required with cuff volumes.

The fixation of an endotracheal tube requires care and there must be no risk that patient movement or coughing will dislodge the tube, which should be tied securely and comfortably with tape. An oral endotracheal tube should be kept away from the corners of the mouth and checks made that the tape is not cutting into the neck. Sores can be avoided by good care of the mouth and lips and by frequently altering the position of the tube. A swivel connector may be used to connect the ventilator tubing firmly to the endotracheal tube. The ventilator tubing or breathing circuit should be well-supported and should not be allowed to drag on the tracheal tube.

When a patient is being turned, one nurse should be responsible for the head of the patient to ensure that there is no pull on the tube. Although the position of the tube in the trachea will have been initially checked by the anaesthetist subsequent movement may alter this, hence both sides of the chest should be checked for correct movement and breath sounds on inspiration and expiration, especially after turning the patient. It is possible for a long endotracheal tube to slip down into a main bronchus and result in ventilation of only one lung (Fig. 10.2).

Although once practised, it is not usual to release the modern low-pressure cuff at intervals as this cannot be expected to reduce damage to the epithelium of the trachea. In addition, this practice may result in under-ventilation or soiling of the trachea with secretions, gastric or pharyngeal fluids or blood. If cuff release is a practice of the unit, it is vital that the pharynx is sucked out and the patient positioned 'head down' before the cuff is released.

Tracheal suction is described in detail on page 187, and should be carried out as often as necessary. Hourly suction should always be performed otherwise inspissation causes the secretions to become more difficult to remove.

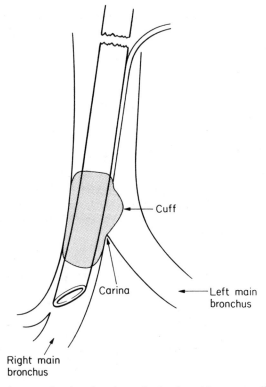

Fig. 10.2 An incorrectly placed endotracheal tube with non-ventilation on the left lung

Tracheostomy

Many aspects of tracheostomy care are similar to the care of the patient with an endotracheal tube. The patient should always be told that a tracheostomy is to be performed, explanation and positive reassurance doing much to ease fears. Likewise after the operation, a confident nurse will be a great comfort to the patient.

Tracheostomy is best carried out as a planned procedure in the operating theatre. On return to the unit, the patient should be observed for signs of oedema, haemorrhage and correct placement of the tube. Suction will be required frequently at first and blood will almost certainly be present in the aspirate, but if bleeding continues or becomes profuse the patient should be seen by a doctor.

The same principles apply for recording cuff size and volume, methods of inflation, fixation and suction as in endotracheal tubes. The tracheostomy tube should be changed every five to seven days. Cuffed tubes are obviously required for patients being ventilated, but may also be indicated where swallowing and laryngeal reflexes are disturbed in spontaneously breathing patients, as fluid or food inhalation is prevented. Many patients will be fed by nasogastric tube but regurgitation can occur and still presents an inhalation danger. As control of swallowing is regained and the laryngeal reflexes return the cuff can be deflated.

Fixation of a tracheostomy tube is easier than an endotracheal tube and is more comfortable for the patient. However, care should be taken when moving the patient, as movement can contribute to the incidence of complications. The intubation tray containing spare sterile tracheostomy tubes and tracheal dilators should always be at hand. The skin around the stoma should be cleansed four-hourly with 0.9 % saline and, if necessary, the tapes securing the tracheostomy tube changed by two nurses, one of whom must be skilled in the procedure. In some units key-hole dressings are applied, to prevent friction between the flange of the tracheostomy tube and the skin. They should be changed if they become moist. Bacteriological swabs should be sent routinely for culture and sensitivity. The neck incision should not have required sutures but any can be removed on the fourth day.

Complications such as haemorrhage and emphysema require the attention of medical staff, who should be summoned without delay if serious trouble is suspected. Dislodgement of the tracheostomy tube (through turning, vigorous coughing or even by the patient himself) is a life-threatening complication and must be dealt with immediately. The urgency is not as great if the patient is breathing spontaneously and the tracheostomy is several days old because the patient will continue to breathe through the established stoma. A new tracheostomy however will close if the tube becomes dislodged and then the following steps must be taken:

1 Send someone to telephone the duty anaesthetist.

2 Place the patient flat with head extended over a pillow.

3 Insert tracheal dilators into the stoma to open it.

4 Insert a sterile tracheostomy tube if possible; if not, keep the tracheostomy open until help arrives and observe the patient's colour; maintain ventilation by manual means if necessary.

The development of a tracheo-oesophageal fistula and severe haemorrhage from erosions of the great vessels is fortunately rare. In the event of the latter, suction, over-inflation of the cuff and a steep head-down position will be of some help until medical assistance arrives.

Changing a temporary tracheostomy tube. An anaesthetist must always perform this aseptic technique the first time the tube is changed. Thereafter it may be carried out by two nurses (one of whom must be proficient in the procedure) who should ensure that medical staff are nearby for immediate assistance, if required.

Procedure for changing a temporary tracheostomy tube

1 Prepare a trolley with the following sterile equipment: a dressing pack; lifting forceps; two tracheostomy tubes (one of the same size and one a size smaller than the patient has *in situ*); tracheostomy tapes (attach to the tubes and inflate the cuffs carefully to test patency); tracheal dilators; a sterile 10 ml syringe; sterile pairs of artery forceps and scissors; sterile disposable gloves; sterile 0.9% saline for cleansing the stoma.

2 Check the suction apparatus.

3 Explain the procedure to the patient and ensure privacy.

4 Position the patient correctly with the head down and neck extended.

5 Wash hands and put on a face mask and sterile gloves.

6 *The assistant* puts on a mask and washes hands, and proceeds with pharyngeal and tracheal suction using an aseptic technique.

7 *The operator* arranges the sterile dressing towel below the tracheostomy site and places on it the tracheal dilators, tracheostomy tubes, artery forceps and syringe.

8 *The operator* cleans the area around the stoma quickly; if the patient has a long-standing tracheostomy and is breathing spontaneously, more time can be taken. Pure oxygen may be inspired for a few breaths before commencing the next stage.

9 *The assistant* disconnects the patient from the ventilator, carefully and quickly cuts the tracheostomy tapes and deflates the cuff.

10 *The operator* inserts the tracheal dilator forceps so that the blades of the instrument are alongside the tube in the trachea and then opens the blades to keep the track open.

11 The assistant then gently removes the tube.

12 The operator immediately replaces a sterile tracheostomy tube and inflates the cuff with the required amount of air.

13 The assistant inflates the lungs manually with an anaesthetic breathing bag or a self-filling inflating bag and checks that the lungs are correctly inflating using a stethoscope. Only then is the patient reconnected to the ventilator and the tapes tied securely.

14 The operator applies a dry tracheostomy dressing, if required, using an aseptic technique.

15 The size of the tube inserted, the date of insertion and the amount of air used to inflate the cuff are recorded. The prescribed F_{IO_2} is again checked.

Closure of a temporary tracheostomy. Signs that the time has come to close the tracheostomy include ability to cough adequately, full control of laryngeal and pharyngeal reflexes, absent or scanty secretions on suction, satisfactory respiratory function and a satisfactory chest X-ray.

Closure is undertaken only on the instructions of the medical staff and must be performed only by a trained nurse who is skilled in the procedure.

Procedure for closing a temporary tracheostomy

1 Prepare a trolley with a dressing pack, sterile 0.9% saline for cleaning the stoma, and two tracheostomy tubes (one of the same size and the other a size smaller than the tube being removed).

2 Check the suction apparatus.

3 Explain the procedure to the patient.

4 Place the patient in a position that is comfortable to him; it is not necessary to lie the patient down with the neck extended.

5 Aspirate the pharynx and trachea, using an aseptic technique.

6 Cut the tracheostomy tapes, deflate the cuff and remove the tube.

7 Aspirate any further secretions expectorated.

8 Clean around the stoma using the basic dressing procedure.

Continued

9 Loosely cover the stoma with dry gauze fixed with adhesive tape; the
   stoma will heal spontaneously. It is incorrect to cover a tracheostomy
   by an occlusive dressing as this does not aid healing and has the
   danger of precipitating interstitial emphysema and cellulitis.

The patient should be observed closely for several hours immediately
following removal of the tube for signs of respiratory distress such as
tachycardia, dyspnoea, drowsiness, sweating and cyanosis. Observation
of the patient's swallowing reflex and encouragement to expectorate
secretions helps to prevent atelectasis. Deep breathing exercises and
speaking are also to be encouraged, and any prolonged hoarseness must
be reported. Initially, only water should be given to the patient to drink
until laryngeal competence is demonstrated. The wound must be
observed for signs of excessive secretions and infection and redressed as
necessary. An identical sterile tube and one a size smaller than the one
removed and a pair of tracheal dilators must be kept at the bedside until
the stoma is closed.

Tracheal suction

The exact type of equipment and the details of the procedure will vary
from hospital to hospital. There are, however, some important principles
to remember concerning suction:

(a) It is a sterile procedure.

(b) If the patient is receiving mechanical ventilation of the lungs, two
nurses are preferable for the procedure.

(c) If the patient is receiving mechanical ventilation of the lungs,
reconnect between each suction.

(d) Use each catheter and glove once only.

(e) The only movement during the withdrawal of the catheter should
be a gentle rolling between the thumb and index finger; never move the
catheter up and down during suction.

(f) Never introduce the catheter while suction is operative at the tip, as
this will damage the mucous membrane.

(g) Care should be taken not to leave the patient disconnected from the
ventilator for too long. A method that has been advocated for avoiding
this is for the nurse to 'hold her breath' at the same time—when the nurse
needs a breath, so will the patient. This is inadvisable; the procedure
should be timed and not last more than 20–30 seconds.

(h) Adequate humidification prevents secretions becoming sticky and
reduces crusting.

(i) Because these patients are prone to infection, specimens of tracheal
aspirate should be sent to the laboratory on alternate days for
examination.

(j) Tenacious secretions may be loosened by instilling 2 ml of 0.9 %
saline just before suction.

Procedure for tracheal suction

1 Prepare the patient by explanation.

2 Check equipment; fill the suction jug with water.

3 Put on a mask.

4 Wash hands.

5 Open a sterile glove and suction catheter.

6 Put on the sterile glove.

7 With the gloved hand, attach the catheter to the Y-connection on the apparatus.

8 Switch on the suction machine using the ungloved hand.

9 Remove the cover from the suction catheter and the connection to the ventilator with the ungloved hand; preferably a second nurse should be available to perform the latter.

10 With the limb of the Y-piece unblocked, introduce the catheter into the tube with the gloved hand until about one inch is left outside; alternatively, introduce the catheter after kinking near the top (Fig. 10.3).

Continued

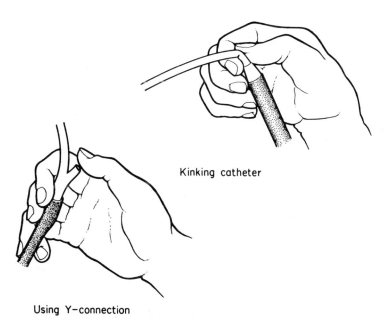

Kinking catheter

Using Y-connection

Fig. 10.3 Tracheal suction

11 Block the limb of the Y-piece or unkink the catheter and withdraw slowly.

12 Reconnect the patient to the ventilator if on IPPV.

13 Clear the suction tubing by applying suction to the water in the jug.

14 Repeat this procedure using a clean catheter and glove on each insertion, connecting the patient to the ventilator between each period of suction.

15 Empty the water jug and dry at the end of each session of suction

16 Wash hands.

Bronchoscopy

This procedure is carried out by a doctor with a nurse assistant who might be required to operate the suction catheter and biopsy forceps and be responsible for maintaining the illumination of the bronchoscope. During the procedure the patient's pulse and respiratory rate should be checked and recorded. Observations are important following bronchoscopy and frequent recordings must be made of the pulse, blood pressure and respiratory state and rate. The sputum, which may be copious, should be observed for persistent bloodstaining.

General care of patients on ventilators

1 *Communication.* An explanation must be given to the patient of all procedures carried out, and of the reason why he cannot speak—that it is not permanent and that he will be able to talk normally after the endotracheal or tracheostomy tube is removed.

If the patient is fully orientated and able, writing materials should be provided with which to communicate with staff and relatives. It is important for nurses to be aware of the patient's needs and orientated with signs such as a raised eyebrow and a closing eye for the very necessary 'yes' or 'no' communication. Where possible a figurative communication board should be provided, such as the alphabet written out so that the patient can point to the letters, thus explaining his needs, or caricature drawings depicting the needs of the patient (a drink, bedpan, etc). Alternative stimulation can be provided by radios, television and books, and relatives should be encouraged to visit.

All staff should always assume that an unconscious patient is able to hear, and therefore great care must be taken by all in what is discussed at the bedside.

2 *The eyes.* In an unconscious or paralysed patient, care of the eyes is vital. The eye reflexes are absent and the cornea is liable to damage, so the

eyes should be swabbed with sterile 0.9 % saline and artificial tears (hypromellose) instilled two-hourly, following inspection, to prevent drying of the cornea. On some units it may be the practice for the eyes to be kept closed by sticking the lids with some form of non-traumatic adhesive tape, such as micropore tape. If there is discharge or inflammation, a swab should be taken for bacteriological examination and chloramphenicol eyedrops (0.5 %) used until the sensitivity is known.

3 *The nose.* This should be cleaned if necessary with cotton wool.

4 *The mouth.* The mouth of any debilitated patient quickly becomes dirty if proper care is not taken. The following two-hourly regimen should be followed:

(a) Remove any dentures.
(b) Clean the mouth thoroughly with a sodium bicarbonate solution; a weak solution of hydrogen peroxide prepared by the pharmacy can be used prior to this, if necessary.
(c) Swab the mouth with a mouthwash, e.g. compound thymol glycerine.
(d) Apply a small amount of glycerine if the mouth is very dry.
(e) Apply soft white paraffin or yellow lanolin liberally around lips.

Systemic antibiotics may result in fungal infections of the mouth and tongue. These can be treated with nystatin mixture applied locally.

5 *The skin.* The patient should be blanket-bathed daily and washed as frequently as necessary. The patient's skin must be left perfectly dry, particularly in the groins and axillae, and great care taken in drying the perineum as it soon becomes red and sore. Regular turning will assist in preserving the skin.

6 *Pressure points.* The most effective way of preventing pressure sores is frequent turning, two-hourly for unconscious or paralysed patients. Pressure points (shoulders, elbows, spine, knees, buttocks, ankles and heels) should be protected, and cream applied if necessary. Every two hours the calf muscles should be massaged to help prevent deep vein thrombosis and passive movements carried out in all limbs. Careful positioning of the limbs is necessary in the paralysed or unconscious patient in order to prevent deformities, and a pillow should be used to keep the knees apart. Ripple beds may prove useful in these patients.

Oxygen therapy

Apart from an emergency situation, oxygen therapy is always prescribed by the medical staff and all nurses should be aware of the importance to the patient of receiving the correct concentration of oxygen. It is important to understand the method by which it is to be given and the oxygen flow rate control of the equipment.

Oxygen masks are disposable and tend to be uncomfortable, but this can be improved in most masks by attending to the stretch of the elastic and by placing cotton wool or padding where the elastic touches the skin. Masks rapidly become soiled and lose shape so they should be changed as required. Alterations to improve comfort must not interfere with the principle of the design. Frequent checks should be made to ensure that the added oxygen is flowing into the mask and reports given of changes in the patient's skin colour, particularly in the colour of the lips.

Chest drainage

Some surgical patients in the unit will have chest drains which require special attention. A simple system of drainage is via a glass tube opening into a glass cylinder under sterile distilled water or 3.8 % citrate, to which has been added sterile antifoam (Fig. 10.4). This allows blood to drain but prevents air from gaining access to the pleural cavity, hence maintaining a negative intrapleural pressure. The drainage can be measured every half to one hour by referring to the calibrations on the cylinder.

Suction, if required, is applied to the other 'short' tube entering the cylinder, using a suction pump to produce a negative pressure of about 3–5 cmH$_2$O (0.3–0.5 kPa). Routine observations include the vacuum setting and the blood volume drainage, at the same time as charting the amount of blood and plasma given intravenously to the patient. The rate of observation depends on the type of case and after open-heart surgery is usually quarter-hourly. In the adult, a continued drainage is excess of 200 ml per hour requires explanation and a doctor should be called.

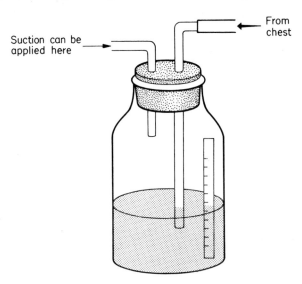

Suction can be applied here

From chest

Fig. 10.4 Chest drainage

Following pulmonary operations there may be air leakage from the lung, the pump suction producing a continual bubbling of air through the fluid in the drainage bottle. This air leakage will gradually diminish and usually ceases within two to three days. Subsequently, it is important to ensure by chest X-ray that the lung remains expanded after the suction has ceased and only after this has been checked should the chest drainage tube be removed.

In some units, it is routine to 'milk' a chest tube which is functioning as a blood drain every 15 minutes. This is best performed by using a specially designed roller.

Drainage bottles are changed according to the unit routine or as necessary. Before the bottle is changed two clamps should be placed, one on the patient's side and one on the bottle side of the connection. After the tubing has been clamped a sterile drainage bottle containing the measured volume of sterile water replaces the dirty drainage bottle. The clamps may then be released to re-establish drainage. This ensures that the drain from within the chest will be closed off during the change of drainage bottle and prevents air entering the pleural space with subsequent lung collapse. The connection, usually of plastic, joining the chest drain to the drainage bottle assembly is always a weak point, and should be checked regularly at both ends.

A drainage bottle should never be raised above the level of the patient's sternum otherwise drainage fluid will run back into the chest. In some units it may be the practice to clamp off the drainage bottle if the patient or bottle is to be moved.

If a chest drain should accidentally become displaced from the chest the following steps should be taken:

(a) Apply pressure to the area.
(b) Summon medical help.
(c) Ensure that the patient is maintaining adequate respirations, and if not then hand ventilate.
(d) Prepare a trolley for the re-insertion of a drain.

When a decision has been made to remove a chest drain the following procedure (requiring two nurses) should be followed.

Procedure for removal of a chest drain

1 Prepare a trolley with a dressing pack, stitch cutter, skin preparation and adhesive plaster.

2 Prepare the patient by explanation, and with analgesics and sedatives.

3 Put on masks.

4 Remove the old dressing and expose the wound.

Continued

5 Both nurses wash hands.

6 Clean the skin around the wound with the skin preparation.

7 If there are local sutures (purse string) around the drain wound, prepare to tie these when the drain is removed.

8 Cut the suture holding the drain.

9 Remove the drain; another nurse at the same time ties the sutures.

10 Place an occlusive dressing over the wound.

A chest X-ray will confirm that the lung is still well expanded and that no air has entered during removal. The patient's respiratory rate and colour should be observed closely following the chest drain removal.

Physiotherapy

Physiotherapy is one of the most important supportive forms of treatment given on the ICU, therefore the physiotherapist has an important role and should be present during medical rounds and involved in discussions regarding progress and treatment. A nurse should always be available to assist during the patient's treatment and should understand the principles of the procedures involved so as to enable treatment to be given at any time during the 24 hours that it is needed, even when a physiotherapist is not available.

Ideally, the physiotherapist visits the patient every four hours during the day, and where possible nursing care should be planned to coincide with physiotherapy. The patient should be prepared beforehand by explanation and given analgesics, sedatives and inhalations of mucolytic agents or bronchodilators if necessary. A nurse is needed to assist the physiotherapist with turning the patient, to give suction as required and to hand-ventilate the patient while the chest is being vibrated. For the patient's advantage, the relationship between the nursing staff and physiotherapist must be friendly and co-operative.

Observations

The general condition of the patient will suggest how frequently observations such as blood pressure, apex heart rate, central venous pressure and temperature should be carried out and charted.

The patient should be observed for signs of inadequate ventilation, the ventilator checked and recordings made at routine intervals, usually every quarter to half hour. These include:

(a) the inflation pressure;
(b) the set tidal/minute volume;
(c) the spirometer reading;

(d) the set ventilation rate, which should be counted for one minute;
(e) the oxygen concentration;
(f) the rate of flow of the oxygen, Entonox and/or air, if applicable;
(g) the temperature and water level of the humidifier;
(h) the temperature of inspired gases just as they enter the patient;
(i) that the ventilator tubing is water-free.

All connections should be tight and the lumens of all tubes patent. The anaesthetist always sets the ventilator and nurses must be familiar with these settings to be aware of any changes that may occur.

Familiarity with the clinical signs of inadequate ventilation and with the resuscitative treatment required is essential. Any suspicion of malfunction of the ventilator must be acted upon immediately, ventilation being taken over manually until the anaesthetist has corrected the fault.

Draining of ventilator tubing

This is part of the hourly routine and if not carried out conscientiously will result in obstruction to the gas flow. Some ventilators have water traps, while in others the tubing must be disconnected and drained. In these cases speed is essential as the patient is not ventilated during this period. The ventilator tubing should be changed daily as it quickly becomes prone to the growth of bacteria, especially *Pseudomonas.*

Humidification

The importance of this has already been dealt with on page 73. The inspired gas temperature at the patient end of the ventilator tubing should ideally be around 35°C and should be checked regularly, if it is being measured. It is necessary to ensure that the temperature of the humidifier is appropriate for the apparatus in use. The water level must be checked regularly and maintained with sterile distilled water, and the humidifier changed daily to help prevent the growth of bacteria.

Sedation and analgesia

All drugs are prescribed by the medical staff and should be given and charted as ordered. It is important that patients in ICUs receive adequate sedation and analgesia and nurses should be able to recognise when patients require sedation, especially those on ventilators. Certain patients need to be paralysed in order to maintain adequate ventilation. Sedatives are given with neuromuscular blocking agents so that patients are not aware of their paralysis. Close observation of the effects of sedative and analgesic drugs upon the circulation and respiration is necessary in case profound and unexpected effects occur.

The cardiovascular system

Intravenous infusions

A nurse's duties regarding infusions should be directed to the following:
(a) checking that the prescribed fluid is administered to the correct patient;
(b) controlling the flow at the prescribed rate;
(c) checking that the container and fluid show no obvious faults or contamination:
(d) observing whether the intravenous line remains patent;
(e) inspecting the site of injection and reporting any abnormality;
(f) observing and reporting on the condition of the patient;
(g) maintaining all necessary records.

All patients following cardiothoracic surgery have both central and peripheral infusions. Other patients in the ICU usually have either a central or a peripheral 'line'. Peripheral veins are not ideal for the infusion of hypertonic fluids and intravenous feeding as they rapidly thrombose. Intravenous infusions containing a vasopressor agent such as adrenaline are always given via a central vein as leakage into superficial tissues may result in necrosis. Since the introduction of three-way taps with extension leads it is possible to give more than one solution into each line, therefore it is necessary to ensure that the solutions are not incompatible with each other.

All solutions must be prescribed by the doctor on the fluid balance chart. Compatibility of blood will require careful checking against the patient's haematology notes together with the haematology form and the patient's identity band. Patients receiving blood should be watched carefully for reactions due to sensitivity or incompatibility such as rashes, pains in the back, rise in temperature and pulse rate.

When using electrolyte solutions, great care must be exercised in checking the strength of solution prescribed since dextrose, saline, sodium bicarbonate, mannitol and similar solutions are all available in various strengths. Two nurses should always check each solution with the doctor's prescription before it is given to the patient.

Microdrip sets with electrically driven pumps or syringes are often used and they are a convenient way of ensuring the correct hourly infusion rate. They should be checked frequently to ensure that the infusion is running at the correct number of drops per minute and the amount of fluid given on the fluid balance chart recorded at the end of each hour. Colour coding on the charts and infusions makes it much easier for both nurses and medical staff to identify when drugs such as adrenaline are being given.

The intravenous catheter should be inserted under strict aseptic conditions, with care being taken to avoid kinking or tension, and covered by a sterile dressing. Occasionally the catheter is stitched into position.

The connections of the administration sets are changed daily or when necessary. Blood filters should be used when giving a blood transfusion. Each unit has its own policy as to whether the infusion site should be inspected and re-dressed daily or less frequently, but the dressing technique must be aseptic at all times. At the first sign of inflammation around the infusion site the drip should be discontinued and taken down and the catheter tip sent for bacteriological culture. Flushing of the cannula may be necessary and can be performed by a nurse who has received the appropriate training.

The addition and administration of drugs via intravenous fluids. All drugs and infusions are prescribed by the medical staff on the appropriate charts. State Registered and Enrolled nurses may administer intravenous drugs or add a drug to an intravenous fluid providing they have received the appropriate hospital training and are competent in the procedure. An aseptic technique must be observed to minimise the possibility of contamination with micro-organisms. It is important that nurses do not give a drug unless perfectly clear about its action on the patient. If in doubt, a doctor should be called, especially if there is an unexpected reaction to the drug. Each unit should have an intravenous additive incompatibility chart available for checking that no warning against adding the drug to the fluid is given.

The legal position of a nurse who performs these duties must be clearly understood by the doctor and the nurse.

Pressure measuring equipment

Central venous pressure (CVP) lines. The measurement of central venous pressure is now a standard procedure in the ICU. A nurse's duty here is similar to the care of infusions—the line must be kept flowing and infection prevented. Accurate readings will be required hourly or even more frequently. From a radio-opaque catheter passed into the right atrium from either an antecubital, subclavian or internal jugular vein, the pressure can be measured by the commercially available CVP measuring sets as shown (Fig. 10.5) or a pressure transducer. A fluid manometer is linked to an intravenous giving set, and to the catheter via a three-way tap. It is mounted on a centimeter scale.

Procedure for Measuring CVP

1 Place the patient in a horizontal position or, if this is not possible, at 45° head-up; the patient should then be placed in the same position for each reading so that valid comparisons can be made.

2 Check that the infusion is running freely, i.e. that the catheter is patent.

Continued

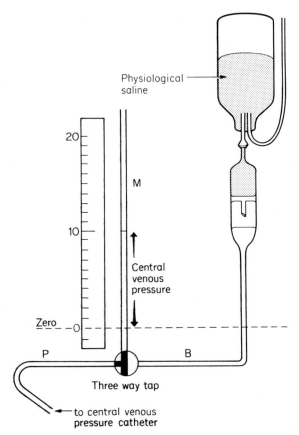

Fig. 10.5 A central venous pressure measuring set

3 Flush the catheter if necessary; this should be carried out only by a nurse who is competent in this procedure.

4 Check zero with a spirit level, using the accepted reference point preferred in the unit; this is usually the sternal angle or the phlebostatic axis (page 49).

5 Turn the tap to allow the fluid to run from the bottle or bag into the measuring column (M).

6 Turn the tap to connect the measuring column to the patient (P) and allow the level to fall; respiratory oscillations should be present.

7 When the level stops falling take the measurement which will be in cmH_2O. This can be converted to mmHg or kPa if necessary (page 9).

8 Turn the tap to connect the patient once more to infusion (B) and set to a slow drip rate to keep the catheter patent.

When a transducer is used, it is attached to the catheter and also linked to a bedside monitor containing an amplifier and an oscilloscope display. The catheter is kept patent by incorporating a continuous flush device between it and the transducer. This method provides a continuous measurement of CVP.

Right atrial (RA) lines. These are used to measure the direct right atrial pressure using either a standard CVP measuring set or a transducer with an incorporated continuous 'flushing' device. The transducer table is aligned to the level of the patient's right atrium (the phlebostatic axis) to obtain an accurate mean RA pressure. The table should be re-aligned when the patient is moved. A nurse's responsibility is the same as with CVP lines—the prevention of infection.

Left atrial (LA) lines. These provide a continuous measurement of left atrial pressure. They are connected to a transducer and then linked to the bedside monitoring system containing a pressure amplifier and an oscilloscope display. The catheter is then kept patent by incorporating a continuous flush device with heparinised saline* between it and the transducer. The transducer table is aligned to the level of the patient's left atrium (the phlebostatic axis) and, as with RA lines, the table must be re-aligned when the patient is moved.

Nurses should be aware of the following special nursing points:
    (a) that the introduction of infection into the line is avoided;
    (b) that no infusions are given through the LA line;
    (c) that no blood samples are taken from a LA line except in specially indicated circumstances;
    (d) that absolutely no air gets into the line (risk of systemic air embolus).

Pulmonary artery (PA) lines (e.g. Swan-Ganz catheters). These are used for the monitoring of pulmonary artery pressure and the indirect left atrial pressure. Some of these catheters also provide the facilities of CVP monitoring and can be used for the administration of intravenous fluids.
    The general principles already enumerated should be observed. There are three types of special catheter:

    (a) *The double-lumen catheter* is used to measure PA and pulmonary capillary wedge pressure (PCWP) and is primarily a monitoring catheter; mixed venous blood from the PA may be sampled.

* 500–1000 i.u. (5–10 mg) heparin per 500 ml 0.9 % NaCl solution.

(b) *The triple-lumen catheter* functions in the same way as the double-lumen catheter but there is an extra (RA) lumen to allow monitoring of CVP and RA pressures and for giving drugs. This additional lumen is useful if emergency drugs are needed and for taking blood samples.

(c) *The thermodilution-catheter* has four separate lumens and allows the functions of the triple-lumen catheter but has an extra lumen containing thermistor wires and opening 4 cm from the catheter tip. Cardiac output can be determined by the thermodilution method.

In the triple and quadruple lumen catheters the distal lumen is attached to a flushing device. The other lumen must be slowly and continually flushed to prevent clotting inside. Blood and hyperalimentation products must not be attached to any of these catheters because of the high risk of sepsis. Medication must be given through the proximal lumen only (never through the distal lumen because very concentrated drugs will damage the endothelium of the PA). Glyceryl trinitrate reacts with polyvinyl chloride (PVC) and should not be given through these catheters.

The infusion tubing attached to PA catheters should be changed every 48 hours and the occlusive dressing to the skin over the point of entry of the catheter changed every 24 hours, after careful cleaning and drying of the skin and tubing.

Pulmonary artery catheters tend to be swept onwards and become unintentionally wedged, with the risk of causing infarction of the lung. A vigorous flush of the catheter in this situation may lead to rupture of the pulmonary vessels, so to avoid this problem PA catheters are sometimes pulled back into a larger trunk of the pulmonary artery and not advanced to a 'wedge' position until such a measurement is next required.

The problem of catheters slipping back into the right ventricule is unusual except in patients with high PA pressures and may lead to extrasystoles being provoked by the tip of the catheter striking the walls of the cavity of the ventricle. In such a situation the balloon may be inflated with 1.5 ml air or CO_2 to protect the tip of the catheter and reduce the risk of extrasystoles, while at the same time medical help may be requested.

Procedure for removing LA, RA and PA catheters

These catheters are removed by a nurse at the doctor' request.

1 Prepare a trolley with a small dressing pack, stitch cutter, Normasol sachet, Polybactrin spray and Airstrip plaster.

2 Prepare the patient by explanation.

3 Position the patient on his back.

4 Wash hands.

5 Clean the area around the line with antiseptic.

6 Cut the skin suture.

7 Remove the catheter, applying counter pressure with a gauze swab.

8 Apply pressure to the site until bleeding stops (usually 3–5 mins).

9 Clean the area with Normasol.

10 Spray the area with Polybactrin.

11 Apply the Airstrip plaster.

A record should be made on the patient's observation chart that the line has been removed and its length. The patient should be observed carefully for signs of localised bleeding and cardiac tamponade.

Arterial lines (cannulae). In the ICU patients have intra-arterial lines inserted for two reasons:

1 to gain continuous and accurate direct measurement of arterial pressure;
2 ease of access for arterial blood samples, therefore avoiding the discomfort of frequent arterial punctures.

The cannulation is carried out by a doctor using an aseptic technique, but the subsequent nursing care of an arterial line is also of vital importance. The cannula must always be firmly secured with strapping (Fig. 10.6), applied over the cannulation site only, care being taken that circulation to

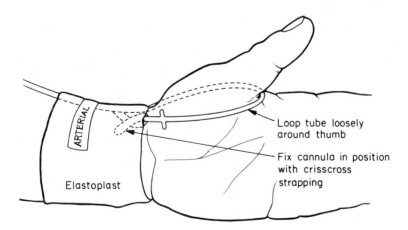

Fig. 10.6 To show how an arterial cannula can be fixed securely in position; note the identifying label

the limb is not impeded. The identity of the arterial line should be made obvious by labelling. Thereafter the site of insertion of the cannula should be redressed daily or as necessary, using an aseptic technique.

The patient's arm should be well supported with the site of insertion and all connections clearly visible, so that any disconnection is immediately detected. The line is usually attached to a continuously flushing device, otherwise it has to be flushed regularly with heparinised saline using a syringe. Arterial lines should be flushed only by a nurse who is skilled in the procedure and gentle pressure with a small volume of solution (1–2 ml) should be used; excessive pressures and volumes can cause retrograde flushing to the level of the carotid arteries. It is important to be aware that no drugs should ever be administered through an arterial line.

The patient's arm and hand should be assessed at frequent intervals for warmth, colour, pain or swelling, and any significant changes should be reported to the medical staff, who should also be informed if the line becomes difficult to flush or if the patient complains of pain in the limb.

Procedure for taking a sample of blood from an arterial line

This should be carried out only by or with the supervision of a nurse who is skilled in the procedure. Great care must be taken to avoid the introduction of air or infection into the artery.

1 Place the appropriate sterile syringes and blood sample bottles by the patient.

2 Wash hands.

3 Withdraw blood into 5 ml syringe from the three-way tap until the line is clear of saline.

4 Attach a sterile syringe to the three-way tap and withdraw the appropriate amount of blood.

5 Flush the line using either the incorporated 'flushing' device or heparinised solution in a syringe until the line is clear of blood.

6 Insert the sample into the appropriate bottles, labelled and attached to the investigation form.

Procedure for the removal of an arterial cannula

These lines are removed by a nurse at a doctor's request.

1 Prepare a trolley with a dressing pack, cleansing solution, antibiotic spray and Elastoplast or other occlusive dressing.

2 Cleanse the area around the cannula and place a gauze swab over the site.

3 Remove the arterial cannula and apply firm pressure over the site for a minimum of five minutes or until the bleeding stops. A 5 ml syringe containing heparinised saline should be attached to the arterial line and aspirated as the cannula is being removed; this often assists in the removal of any intra-arterial clots that may be present.

4 Spray the site with antibiotic spray.

5 Dress the site with a sterile dry dressing using a non-touch technique.

6 Apply strapping.

7 Leave the patient lying comfortably with the site exposed.

Following this procedure, check the hand at frequent intervals for warmth, colour and swelling. the doctor must be informed if the hand and forearm become discoloured or swollen, if the patient complains of pain in the limb or if there is haematoma formation.

ECG leads

The majority of electrodes used for ECG monitoring are now of the disposable adhesive disc pattern and therefore suitable for long-term monitoring. They are changed routinely or as necessary depending upon the quality of the electrode contact.

The quality of the ECG trace depends upon the contact of the skin with the electrodes, hence it is most important that the skin is prepared effectively, the hair under the disc shaved and the area cleaned. This repetitive skin preparation can cause the patient some discomfort so the electrodes should not be replaced over their original site if possible.

Metal plates. These are still used in some countries for limb leads. Electrode jelly is used liberally to establish electrical contact then the plates are secured by rubber straps, which should never be too tight. The straps and plates must be removed immediately after use and cleaned and dried before being placed on the next patient. The electrode jelly should be removed from the patient's skin.

Pacemaker leads

A nurse's duty with relation to pacemaker leads is to ensure that they do not become disconnected or touch one another. Internal pacing is commonly carried out in the ICU, usually by a catheter introduced into the heart via a peripheral vein under radiographic control or by epicardial leads placed at operation. The pacing leads may be a temporary measure until the conducting mechanism of the heart recovers, or until a permanent pacemaker can be inserted. The record and observation charts should contain the rate of pacing and this should be checked against the ECG to ensure that pacing is maintained. If pacing control is lost, the doctor in charge of the case should be informed.

Intra-aortic balloon counterpulsation (IABC). The use of this cardiac assist device is becoming more frequent, both in Coronary Care and Cardio-thoracic Units. The IABC is inserted using an aseptic technique by the medical staff, then a chest X-ray is taken to ensure that the catheter is in the correct position.

Nurses should be fully aware and understand the indications for balloon counterpulsation and the effect that it will have upon the patient's condition and observations. The subsequent nursing care and observations are of vital importance.

Since an ECG signal is required to activate the machine, it is important that the skin contact for the electrodes is reliable. The directly measured arterial blood pressure must be constantly monitored in order to confirm that the balloon counterpulsation is appropriately timed within the cardiac cycle. The timing of the IABC will need adjusting if there is a significant change in the heart rate or rhythm, as its effect relies upon accurate and consistent timing in relation to the heart action. Other parameters which should be recorded are the patient's systolic blood pressure, pulse rate, left atrial pressure or wedge pressure, the IABC augmentation ratio (1:1, 1:2, 1:3 etc.), cardiac rhythm and the balloon filling pressure.

The patient should be nursed in a comfortable position, ensuring that there is no tension exerted on the balloon catheter. The presence of the balloon conduit in the femoral artery produces partial obstruction of that vessel and consequently a certain amount of impaired circulation to the involved extremity. It is vitally important therefore that the arterial supply to the leg is continually assessed.

Immediately after taking over the management of these patients, it is a nurse's duty to assess the status of the leg and foot and, particularly, to make an assessment of the pulses in that extremity. An indication should be made on the observation chart as to whether the pulses are present or not. Thereafter any significant changes in these pulses, cooling of the extremity or colour changes must be reported to the surgeon immediately.

Gas leaks can occur in the system. Various IABC systems use different gases, usually helium or carbon dioxide, to inflate the balloon. Should leaks occur, nurses must be familiar with the procedures for correcting the problem. Most leaks are of a non-recurring nature, and require nothing more than refilling the system with the appropriate gas medium.

Emergency re-opening of the chest

This procedure requires the presence of at least two nurses (one of whom must be familiar with the situation) to assist the surgeons and the anaesthetist and to provide the appropriate equipment and drugs. The drugs, dosage and time given and, in the case of cardiac arrest, the number of DC shocks and joules delivered must be recorded. Where possible, observation and charting of the patient's blood pressure and apex rate should be continued.

Following the procedure, the patient's consciousness level should be observed frequently and the patient's physiological observations recorded quarter-hourly. The relatives should be informed of the patient's condition.

Cardiac arrest

The details of the treatment of cardiac arrest are given on page 21. Nurses should be able to institute the cardiac arrest drill and be able to give external defibrillation if necessary. Obviously this responsibility can be given only to fully instructed staff. External cardiac massage is something that every nurse must know and perform efficiently, and the cardiac arrest drill must be perfect in the unit. Patients should be nursed on boards or on beds with a hard surface. Each patient should have the equipment for manual ventilation with oxygen attached beside the bed and nurses should be familiar with the operation of such an assembly.

Accurate records of each cardiac arrest must be kept, with particular reference to the drugs used. During arrest drill, nursing staff must keep calm even when confronted with a barrage of simultaneous requests from the doctors present and, above all, be familiar with the arrest equipment and ready with the commonly used drugs.

In the ICU, the resuscitation trolley should contain equipment for intravenous infusion, a selection of drugs and a defibrillator (see Appendix II). A bronchoscope should be available for emergency use, and defibrillators, pacemakers, ECG monitors and ventilators available as part of the standard equipment at hand on the unit.

The renal system

Peritoneal dialysis

Nursing staff will be expected to assist in the setting up of peritoneal dialysis and maintain careful observations once established (see page 109). The trolley and bedside requirements are shown in Table 10.1.

During dialysis, accurate observations of pulse, blood pressure, respiration, CVP and temperature are necessary, and accurate volumetric fluid balance and peritoneal dialysis charts must be kept.

Uraemic patients are particularly susceptible to infections, hence strict asepsis is vital. The catheter dressing must be kept dry and frequent mouth and pressure area care carried out. Patients should be turned two-hourly, if immobile, receive regular physiotherapy and be encouraged to

Table 10.1   Requirement for peritoneal dialysis

Trolley	Bedside
large dressing pack	Dialaflex solution and warming tank
3 peritoneal dialysis cannulae	peritoneal dialysis Y-type giving set
sterile artery forceps	infusion stand
Bard Parker scalpel handle and	bucket
No. 15 blade	1 litre jug
suture pack and needle	sterile dressing scissors, in Hibitane
2 ml syringe and hypodermic needle	0.5 %
(lumbar puncture needle if the	heparin, 1000 units in 1 ml potassium
patient is obese)	a selection of needles and syringes
local anaesthetic eg. Lignocaine 1 %	drug added labels
cleansing lotion	masks
razor	disposable gloves
plaster and dressings	specimen pot
	laboratory forms
	peritoneal dialysis chart

breathe deeply as they are susceptible to chest infections. High calorie and protein drinks and diet should be encouraged when applicable. Nurses must follow the doctor's orders regarding the patient's fluid intake, weighing the patient twice daily at the end of a drain cycle. Analgesics may be required for pain relief and should be given as necessary.

Various complications of peritoneal dialysis are indicated in Table 10.2. Any of these complications should be reported to the doctor immediately.

Arterio-venous shunt

An arterio-venous shunt is virtually an extension of the circulatory system and is therefore extremely vulnerable. Correct care of the shunt is vital to ensure that it remains safe, patent and free from infection, otherwise unnecessary complications with potentially fatal results may occur. Meticulous care begins immediately following insertion of the shunt.

Micropore tape must be applied over the joint of the two silastic sections and be 'hemmed' (folded back on itself for easy opening, as with Sellotape) to allow for easy removal. A crepe bandage is used to cover the whole length of the shunt limb to prevent oedema. Labelling of the arterial side of the shunt with red tape should be undertaken only by an SRN with experience in dialysis or haemoperfusion. Two shunt clips should be clipped to the outside layer of the dressing at all times. Check that no kinks are present in the shunt tubing as this results in restricted flow. The insertion site and limb must be observed for signs of haematoma and oedema. It is imperative that any sign of clotting should be reported immediately so that appropriate action may be taken.

Table 10.2 Complications of peritoneal dialysis

---

1 Improper drainage or non-return of fluid caused by:
   (a) misplaced catheter
   (b) kinked catheter
   (c) blocked catheter—in which case the catheter is syringed out with heparinised saline
   (d) dehydrated patient
   (e) patient changing position
2 Pain caused by:
   (a) 6.36% solution being used (as opposed to 1.36%)
   (b) the dialysis solution being too hot or too cold (peritoneal dialysis fluid is always warmed to 30°C.)
   (c) peritonitis, which should not occur if strict asepsis is carried out
3 Leakage around the catheter site
4 Turbid drained dialysate with or without pyrexia (usually an indication of peritonitis)
5 Blood in the dialysate which occurs sometimes initially (major haemorrhage is rare)
6 Dehydration
7 Hyper/hypokalaemia
8 Catheter falling out
9 Hyperglycaemia
10 Cardiac arrest

A patent shunt is recognised by observing the following three points:

1 Red blood must be flowing; if the blood is dark and separating, clotting must be suspected.

2 A pulse must be present; this may be felt by holding the shunt tubing between two fingers (NB *not* thumb and finger). If it is not felt, it may be heard when using a stethoscope placed over the arterial insert.

3 Warmth must be present; a cool shunt indicates very poor or absent flow.

The shunt should be dressed daily (more frequently) if there is any discharge using an aseptic technique. Displaced dressings require immediate replacement. An aseptic technique should always be used when taking blood from a patient's shunt.

Haemofiltration. This is a new development involving the filtration of whole blood through a highly water-permeable membrane. The water molecules are forced out taking with them other, ofter larger, molecules. The process enables the patient to be treated continuously, hence the effects are much less severe than haemodialysis.

Bladder drainage

Bladder catheterisation is required in the unconscious or sedated patient, who will not have control of bladder function, and in the severely ill patient, for whom accurate regular records of urinary output will detect early evidence of pre-renal or renal failure and fluid imbalance. Catheterisation must be carried out as a sterile procedure to prevent infection of the bladder and urinary tract.

Procedure for catheterisation

1 Prepare a trolley with the following sterile equipment: a catheterisation pack, gloves, two towels, a self-retaining catheter, a drainage bag and tubing, water and a syringe, antiseptic solution and adhesive plasters.

2 Inform the patient and explain the procedure.

3 Assist the doctor if the patient is male, because there may be difficulty in passing the catheter; female patients are usually catheterised by the nurse.

4 Position the patient correctly with the heels together and knees apart.

5 Wash hands and put on the sterile gloves.

6 Place one sterile towel over the nearest thigh and the other under the vulva or penis.

7 Place the kidney dish containing the catheter into position between the patient's legs.

8 If the patient is female, separate the labia and swab the vulva with antiseptic lotion. If male, retract the prepuce to the base of the penis and swab the glans penis with antiseptic lotion.

9 Insert the catheter aseptically into the urethra with the free hand, allowing the urine to drain into the kidney dish.

10 Inflate the balloon of the catheter with the correct volume of sterile water and attach the catheter to the drainage tube and bag.

11 Fix the catheter to the patient's thigh, leaving enough slack for movement.

12 Leave the patient dry and comfortable; in female patients the labia should be dried from the centre outwards using the remaining cotton wool.

The amount of urine drained should be measured and tested. If requested samples may be sent for microscopy, culture and biochemical investigation. Urine should never be allowed to contaminate the hands.

In most patients, the hourly urine output must be measured and charted. The urine should be tested for protein, sugar and blood every 4–6 hours and the urinary drainage bag and the jug used for draining the bag should be changed every 24 hours, each patient having his or her own jug. Catheter specimens of urine should be sent on alternate days for culture.

The genitalia of catheterised patients must be cleaned twice daily and be kept dry. Catheters should not be left *in situ* for longer than necessary.

The gastrointestinal tract

An oesophagogastric tube such as Ryle's tube may be required either to keep the stomach empty or for feeding. As there is often difficulty in passing this tube in the already intubated patient, it is best passed at the same time as endotracheal intubation.

Tube feeding

The position of the tube can be checked by testing the aspirate with litmus paper for an acid reaction. If there is no aspirate, the tube can be checked by injecting air—one nurse slowly injects a small amount of air into the tube while a second nurse (who must be an SRN) listens with a stethoscope over the upper left side of the abdomen for the 'gurgling' sound as the air enters the stomach, then the air which has been injected should be withdrawn.

The feed, particularly for babies, should be slightly warmed, free from lumps and allowed to flow in slowly under gravity. The amount and type should be charted. A little water run in to the tube at the end of the feed will help to keep the tube clear. Before each feed the stomach is aspirated and the doctor should be informed if these aspirates are still large in volume, indicating that there is non-absorption. Salivation will be increased by tube feeding, therefore frequent mouth care is vital.

The introduction of fine-bore nasogastric tubes which can be attached to a feeding system (e.g. Clinifeed System 3) allows patients to receive continuous nasogastric feeds, and are much more comfortable than the larger gastric tubes.

Gastric aspiration

Gastric aspiration is an important part of the treatment during ileus. Hourly aspirations may be necessary until bowel activity resumes and the volume of the aspirate must always be charted on the fluid balance chart.

Nasogastric tubes tend to stimulate swallowing, the air swallowed often causing distension and discomfort. Therefore they are often best left to drain into a bag so that air can also escape.

General considerations

Patient morale and support

Mortality rates are higher in an ICU than on a general ward and this can have a demoralising effect on nursing staff. However, a good working atmosphere with a high morale does much to combat this. Close personal involvement with the patient is inevitable. In such a unit it is difficult for a nurse to detach herself emotionally from the patient she nurses through a critical illness. The ability to look at the successes achieved rather than the failures is a great asset and should be emphasised in teaching.

The strain of working with extremely ill patients can be lessened by good working relationships with other members of the hospital staff, whether doctors, physiotherapists or medical social workers. If a nurse feels that she can turn to others for help at any time and rely on them for support, the work will not impose too great an emotional strain. It is most important that one doctor should be in overall administrative charge of the unit, so that the nursing staff feel that they are supported and represented at committee level. The morale of nurses is quickly appreciated by patients, who will be aware of any tension or 'atmosphere' among the staff.

There is no doubt that patients realise the implication of finding themselves in a special ward surrounded by sophisticated equipment and lacking the companionship of the general ward. A great deal of positive reassurance is required with explanation of any procedure in simple language. Above all the patient must be treated as the most important person in the room. Frivolous discussion must be avoided as casual remarks concerning the patient's progress may cause great distress, and it must be remembered that even the apparently unconscious patient may hear and understand what is said. This particularly applies to patients on mechanical ventilation, who may be very alert mentally and will appreciate hearing about the time, the weather or news even if they cannot answer. It is a good practice to address remarks or explanations to patients even if they appear to be unconscious.

Visitors give a feeling of contact with the outside world but should be restricted to the close family. Even then, for the seriously ill patient, visiting should be limited. Staff should always be prepared to talk to visitors and give comfort and advice. Explanation and some idea of the prognosis should be given by the doctors most concerned with the patient.

The medical social worker can be of help, particularly as the patient improves, by offering advice on financial and other matters which nursing staff are not trained to give.

Nursing establishment

The care of patients in the Intensive Care Unit is totally dependent upon the availability of sufficient numbers of trained staff, especially nurses. To provide the essential constant care and attention for each patient, the number of nurses required is based on the ratio of one nurse per patient for each 'shift' throughout the 24 hours. Allowances are also made for holidays and sick leave.

The establishment should be reviewed regularly and at any time when there is a change in the number of working hours or in the holiday entitlement.

Record charts

Each unit will have record charts to suit its own requirements. The design, type and size therefore vary from unit to unit. The charts in the ICU are different from those in the general wards because of the greater number of observations that need to be recorded.

Each unit has its own basic charts for general observations, results, fluid balance, drug and fluid prescriptions. Others should be available for any special observations such as neurological data and peritoneal dialysis. The charts should be filled in neatly so that they represent a clear picture to all concerned with the patient's care. These records play a part in maintaining a check on the patient's routine treatment and the effects of drug administration.

The frequency of observations depends upon the severity of the patient's clinical condition, but it is unlikely that observations ever need recording more than quarter-hourly. Frequent observations will disturb and sometimes tire a patient and interrupt general nursing care so, where possible, the patient should be left undisturbed at night.

Responsibilities and training

The responsibilities of nurses in the ICU are great and manifold. The work must be taken conscientiously and seriously, problems of personal life being left outside the unit door. A nurse's prime duty is towards the patient. Doctors' instructions must be carried out precisely but not blindly and nurses must feel free to approach the doctors for explanations. Observation is paramount and training should be directed towards the early detection of abnormalities whether in the patient's colour, pulse rate or ECG, or in the more general aspects of the patient's appearance.

The care of critically-ill patients demands the highest standards of nursing care and skill, therefore nurses wishing to work in the specialised field of intensive care must be trained accordingly. Training is of two types—either a recognised formalised course, such as JBCNS 100 in General Intensive Care, or 'In-Service Training'.

In-service training is a continuous and informal process of learning designed to introduce student nurses to the policies and practices of the hospital, unit and work situation. It should also provide up-dating on clinical, organisational and professional matters. Alternatively, training by the specialised course includes a more formal educational programme over a set period of time, with assessment at intervals throughout the course, and the award of a certificate of proficiency to successful students at the end.

Both 'in-service' and 'course' nurses will need constant close supervision initially, hence there should always be enough senior staff on duty to guarantee that safe nursing practices and an established standard of nursing care are constantly maintained. The experience and confidence to be gained during this time is invaluable, and student nurses should emerge confident enough to deal with any intensive care situation that may occur with a firm basis of physiological understanding.

Appendix I

Usual doses of drugs commonly used in the Intensive Care Unit

For simplicity many of the drug doses quoted in this text are for an adult of 70 kg body weight—the so-called 'physiological' adult.

The ideal drug dosage is that dose which is enough to produce for the patient the optimal therapeutic effect with the least possible amount of the drug. In practice an average dose is used, but even apparently identical patients do not respond uniformly to exactly the same dose of drug. The calculated average dose is simply a starter and subsequent doses are adjusted according to the patient's response. This is particularly evident in the case of drugs which exert profound actions on the cardiovascular, respiratory and nervous systems as the starter dose may be enough to cause unwanted effects (e.g. depression of these systems) at the outset. Many drugs are cumulative in the body and patients in ICUs may not be able to eliminate drugs in the way that healthy people can. Interactions between drugs are also of major concern and the list of possible interactions is a formidable one. Again, patients who are critically ill may be especially at risk should interactions between drugs occur.

Children and adults differ in many ways including the metabolism of drugs. The younger the child the greater is the importance of metabolic deficiencies associated with immaturity, for instance neonates are especially sensitive to non-depolarising muscle relaxants (e.g. curare-like drugs). There is no simple rule entirely satisfactory for producing an exact fraction of a known adult dose for administration to a child. Drug dosage is commonly related to body weight although correlations with surface area are more accurate as this parameter relates more closely to normal metabolic and physiological processes; this is particularly the case in children. The Dubois nomogram (Fig. A.1) enables surface area to be calculated from measurements of height and weight. In general, children require a higher dose per kilogram body weight than adults (usually twice the adult figures up to 4 months, one and a half times the adult figure up to 7 years), since they have a higher metabolic rate. A common problem is the child who is grossly overweight for his age and height. Calculation by body weight would result in a much larger dose than is really required. In such a case the dose should be calculated from an ideal weight obtained from a table relating height and age.

The average body surface area of a 70 kg adult is about 1.8 m². Thus to calculate the dose for a child the following formula may be used:

$$\frac{\text{approximate dose}}{\text{for patient}} = \frac{\text{surface area of patient (m}^2)}{1.8} \times \text{adult dose}$$

This method is only approximate and does not relate to preterm infants.

Sensitivity or allergy to drugs is now very common and the fact must be noted clearly on the front of the patient's 'notes' and on the treatment card. A 'sensitivities' card is also a useful warning by the patient's bedside to alert the many medical and nursing personnel who are involved in the patient's care.

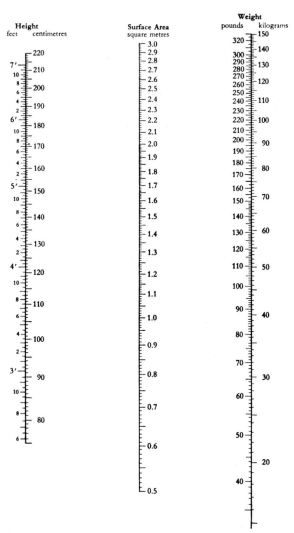

Fig. A.1 Nomogram for the determination of body surface area from height and weight. (From the formula of Dubois and Dubois, *Arch. intern. Med.*, **15**. 868, 1915; $\log S = 0.425 \ \log W + 0.725 \ \log H + 1.8564$; $S =$ body surface in m^2, $W =$ weight in kg, $H =$ height in cm)

Table A.1 Selected Drug doses

SC = subcutaneous;   IV = intravenous; IVI = intravenous infusion;
IM = intramuscular;   SL = sublingual;   PO = by mouth.
Proprietary names in brackets.

Drugs acting on the cardiovascular system

Metaraminol (Aramine)	SC, IM 2–10 mg
	IVI 15–100 mg in 500 ml 0.9 % NaCl or dextrose
Isoprenaline (Isuprel, Saventrine IV)	IVI 0.5–10 μg/min adjusted as required
	After cardiopulmonary bypass, IVI 5–30 μg/min
Adrenaline	Acute anaphylaxis, SC or IM 0.5–1 mg
	Bronchospasm, as a single dose SC or IM 200–500 μg
	After cardiopulmonary bypass, IVI 2.5–20 μg/min
Dobutamine (Dobutrex)	For inotropic action:
	IVI 2.5–10 μg/kg/min, adjusted as required
Dopamine (Intropin)	For inotropic action:
	IVI 5–20 μg/kg/min, increased if necessary
Noradrenaline (Levophed)	IVI 8–12 μg/min, adjusted as required
Methoxamine (Vasoxine)	IM 5–20 mg
	Slow IV 5–10 mg
Phenylephrine	SC, IM 5 mg
	Slow IV 100–500 μg
	IVI 5–20 mg, adjusted as required
Phentolamine (Rogitine)	IV 2.5–10 mg, repeated as necessary
	IVI 5–60 mg over 10–30 minutes at a rate of 0.1–2 mg/min
Sodium nitroprusside (Nipride)	IVI 1 μg/kg/min initially, then adjusted. Rates above 1.5 μg/kg/min should alert to risk of cyanide toxicity
Isosorbide dinitrate	IVI 2–7 mg/h
Glyceryl trinitrate (Tridil or nitroglycerin)	IVI 10–200 μg/min (PVC material is unsuitable for infusion apparatus)
Hydralazine hydrochloride (Apresoline)	Slow IV or IVI 20–40 mg, repeated as necessary
Labetalol hydrochloride (Trandate)	IV 50 mg over 1 minute, repeated after 5 minutes if necessary
	IVI 2 mg/min to a maximum of 200 mg
Practolol (Eraldin)	Slow IV 5 mg, repeated after 5 minutes if necessary

Table A.1 (*Cont.*)

Propanolol	IV 0.5–1 mg over 1 minute, preceded by atropine sulphate 1–2 mg
Lignocaine hydrochloride	Bolus IV 50–100 mg, repeated after 5 minutes if necessary; maintenance, 1–4 mg/min IVI
Mexiletine hydrochloride	IV 100–250 mg over 5–10 minutes, followed by 250 mg IVI as 0.1 % solution over 1 hour, 125 mg/h IVI for 2 hours, then 500 μg/min
Streptokinase (Kabikinase, Streptase)	250 000–600 000 i.u. IVI over 30 minutes, then 100 000 i.u. every hour for up to 1 week
Phenytoin sodium	For ventricular dysrhythmia:
	IV 250 mg at rate not exceeding 50 mg/min, repeated after 10 minutes if necessary
	For status epilepticus:
	IV 250 mg at rate not exceeding 50 mg/min, repeated after 30 minutes if necessary
Disopyramide (Rhythmodan, Norpace)	For ventricular dysrhythmia:
	Slow IV 2 mg/kg to a maximum of 150 mg with ECG monitoring; maintenance, 400 μg/kg/h IVI
Procaine amide hydro-chloride (Pronestyl)	For ventricular dysrhythmia:
	IV 100 mg every 5 minutes with ECG monitoring until dysrhythmia is controlled; maximum dose 1 g; maintenance 0.25–2 mg/min IVI
Verapamil hydrochloride (Cordilox)	For supraventricular tachycardia:
	Slow IV 1.5 mg, repeated after 5–10 minutes if necessary
	IVI 5–10 mg over 1 hour, maximum 100 mg in 24 hours
Digoxin (Lanoxin)	For rapid digitalisation:
	PO 1 mg over 24 hours in divided doses
	IV 0.75–1.25 mg initially then 250 μg every 4 hours under ECG control
Lanatoside C (Cedilanid)	PO 1–1.5 mg daily until digitalised then 250–750 μg daily

Drugs acting on the gastrointestinal system

Metoclopramide hydro-chloride (Maxolon, Primperan)	IM or IV up to 10 mg

Table A.1 (*Cont.*)

Cimetidine (Tagamet)	Slow IV 200 mg every 4–6 hours
	IVI 100–150 mg/h (or 2 mg/kg/h) for 2 hours, repeated after an interval of 4–6 hours; the average infusion rate should not exceed 75 mg/h over 24 hours; maximum dose 2 g daily
	Reduce dose in impaired renal function; caution in hepatic disease; avoid IV injection in high dosage or in cardiovascular impairment (infusion is preferable to minimise dysrhythmias)
Ranitidine (Zantac)	PO 150 mg twice daily; *child* over 8 years, up to 150 mg twice daily. Check acidity of stomach contents with Universal Indicator paper.
	Slow IV 50 mg every 6–8 hours
	IVI 25 mg/hr for 2 hours, repeated if necessary after interval of 6–8 hours.

Drugs acting on the respiratory system

Doxapram (Dopram)	Slow IVI 0.5–4 mg/min
Aminophylline	Slow IV over a period of at least 10–15 minutes, 250–500 mg
Salbutamol (Ventolin)	IV 250 μg every 4 hours
	IVI 3–20 μg/min
Terbutaline sulphate	SC, IM or slow IV 250–500 μg 2–4 times daily; *child* 2–15 years 10 μg/kg to a maximum of 300 μg
	IVI 1.5–5 μg/min for 8–10 hours; reduce dose for children
Naloxone hydrochloride (Narcan)	To antagonise respiratory depressant effects of morphine-like drugs:
	SC, IM, IV 400 μg repeated once or twice at intervals of 2–3 minutes if necessary; *child* 5–10 μg/kg

Drugs acting on the nervous system

Codeine phosphate	IM up to 30 mg when necessary
Pethidine hydrochloride	SC, IM 25–100 mg; *child* IM up to 1 year 1–2 mg/kg, 1–5 years 12.5–25 mg, 6–12 years 25–50 mg
	Slow IV 20–50 mg

Table A.1 (*Cont.*)

Morphine hydrochloride, sulphate or tartrate	SC, IM, 10–20 mg; IV 2.5 mg; *child* up to 1 month 150 μg/kg, 1–12 months 200 μg/kg, 1–5 years 2.5–5 mg, 6–12 years 5–10 mg
Papaveretum (Omnopon)	SC, IM, 10–20 mg every 4 hours; IV 2.5–5 mg
	Note: contains anhydrous morphine 50 % as hydrochloride with the hydrochlorides of other opium alkaloids; 10 mg papaveretum is equivalent in morphine content to 6.25 mg morphine sulphate and not 10 mg as is commonly supposed
Buprenorphine (Temgesic)	SL 200–400 μg every 6–8 hours
	IM or slow IV 300–600 μg every 6–8 hours (Buprenorphine is not antagonised by naloxone)
Phenoperidine (Operidine)	With assisted respiration 2–5 mg, then 1 mg as required; *child* 100–150 μg/kg
Chlorpheniramine maleate (Piriton)	SC, IM, slow IV 5–10 mg to a maximum of 40 mg in 24 hours
Promethazine (Phenergan)	Deep IM, up to 50 mg; much reduced doses in children
Neostigmine methylsulphate (Prostigmin)	Treatment of myasthenia gravis:
	SC, IM, IV 1–2.5 mg at suitable intervals; *child,* neonate 50–250 μg every 4 hours, older children 200–500 μg daily in divided doses
Pyridostigmine bromide (Mestinon)	PO 0.3–1.2 g daily in divided doses at suitable intervals; *child,* neonate 5–10 mg every 4 hours, older children 10 mg initially, increased by 5 mg amounts according to response
	SC, IM, IV 2–5 mg daily; *child,* neonate 200–400 μg every 4 hours, older children initially 0.25–1 mg increasing according to response
Diazepam (Valium, Diazemuls)	IV or slow IV injection, in acute muscle spasm, 2.5–10 mg repeated if necessary after 4 hours; *child,* 100–200 μg/kg repeated if necessary
	IV, tetanus, 100–300 μg/kg repeated every 1–4 hours
	Status epilepticus, convulsions due to poisoning:
	Slow IV 0.5 % solution 150–250 μg/kg at a rate of 0.5 ml (2.5 mg) per 30 seconds, repeated if necessary after 30–50 minutes.

Table A.1 (*Cont.*)

Clonazepam (Rivotril)	Status epilepticus:
	Slow IV or IVI 1 mg over 30 seconds; *child* all ages 500 μg (hypotension and apnoea may occur)
Chlormethiazole edisylate (Heminevrin)	Status epilepticus:
	IVI 0.8 % solution 40–100 ml (320–800 mg) at a rate of 60–150 drops per minute
Lignocaine hydrochloride	Status epilepticus:
	Slow IVI 200–300 mg/h as a 0.2 % solution
	Bolus IV 30 mg, repeated according to the patient's needs
Dantrolene sodium (Dantrium)	For the treatment of malignant hyperpyrexia:
	IV 1 mg/kg initially and repeated if necessary up to a cumulative dose of 10 mg/kg

Drugs acting on infections
Penicillins

Benzylpenicillin (Crystapen, Crystapen G)	IM 300–600 mg, 2–4 times daily; *child* up to 12 years, 10–20 mg/kg daily; neonate 30 mg/kg daily
	IVI up to 24 g daily
Cloxacillin (Orbenin)	IM 500 mg every 4–6 hours
	IV 0.5–1 g every 4–6 hours
	Child, any route $\frac{1}{4}$–$\frac{1}{2}$ adult dose
Flucloxacillin (Floxapen)	IM 250 mg every 6 hours
	Slow IV 250–500 mg every 6 hours
	Child, any route $\frac{1}{4}$–$\frac{1}{2}$ adult dose
Methicillin (Celbenin)	IM or slow IV 1 g every 4–6 hours
Amoxycillin (Amoxil)	IM 500 mg every 8 hours; *child* 50–100 mg/kg daily in divided doses
	IV or IVI 1 g every 6 hours; *child* 50–100 mg/kg daily in divided doses
Ampicillin (Penbritin)	IM or IV 500 mg every 4–6 hours; higher doses in meningitis; *child* any route $\frac{1}{2}$ adult dose
Ampiclox	Ampicillin 250 mg and cloxacillin 250 mg (both as sodium salts) per vial:
	IM or IV 1–2 vials every 4–6 hours; *child* up to 2 years $\frac{1}{4}$ adult dose, 2–10 years $\frac{1}{2}$ adult dose
Ampiclox Neonatal	Ampicillin 30 mg (as trihydrate), cloxacillin 25 mg (as sodium salt) per vial:
	IM or IV, 1 vial (= 75 mg) every 8 hours

Table A.1 (*Cont.*)

Magnapen	Ampicillin 250 mg (as trihydrate) and fluclo-xacillin 250 mg (as sodium salt); 500 mg powder (represents equal amounts of the two ingredients) per vial:
	IM or IV 1 vial every 6 hours; *child* up to 2 years $\frac{1}{4}$ adult dose, 2–10 years $\frac{1}{2}$ adult dose; doses may be doubled in severe infections (double strength vial of 1 g available)
Mezlocillin (Baypen)	IV 2 g every 6–8 hours
	IVI in serious infections 5 g every 6–8 hours
	IM 1–2 g
Azlocillin (Securopen)	Infections due to *Pseudomonas aeruginosa*:
	IV 2 g every 8 hours
	IVI in serious infections 5 g every 8 hours
Carbenicillin (Pyopen)	Infections due to *Pseudomonas aeroginosa* and *Proteus* species:
	Slow IV or rapid IVI, systemic infections, 5 g every 4–6 hours; *child* 250–400 mg/kg daily in divided doses
	IMI urinary tract infections, 2 g every 6 hours; *child* 50–100 mg/kg daily in divided doses
Ticarcillin (Ticar)	Infections due to *Pseudomonas* and *Proteus* species:
	IM or slow IV or rapid IVI 15–20 g daily in divided doses
Mecillinam (Selexidin)	Active against Gram negative organisms, especially enteric bacteria e.g. *Salmonella* species
	Slow IM or IV 5–15 mg/kg every 6–8 hours
Cephalosporins Cefotaxime (Claforan)	IM or IV 1 g every 12 hours; in severe infections up to 12 g in 3–4 divided doses; *child* 100–150 mg/kg daily in 2–4 divided doses; in severe infections, up to 200 mg/kg daily. In severe renal impairment, doses to be halved
	IVI 1–2 g over 20–60 minutes
Cefoxitin (Mefoxin)	IM, IV or IVI 1–2 g every 8 hours; *child* over 2 years 80–150 mg/kg daily in divided doses

Table A.1 (*Cont.*)

Cefuroxime (Zinacef)	IM or IV 750 mg every 8 hours
	IV or IVI in severe infections 1.5 g every 6–8 hours
	Child 30–100 mg/kg daily in divided doses
Cephaloridine (Ceporin)	IM or IV 0.5–1 g every 8–12 hours; maximum 6 g daily; *child* 20–40 mg/kg daily in divided doses, maximum 4 g daily
Cephalothin (Keflin)	IV or IVI 1 g every 4 hours; maximum 12 g daily; *child* 12.5–25 mg/kg every 6 hours
Cephamandole (Kefadol)	IM, IV or IVI 0.5–2 g every 4–8 hours; *child* 50–100 mg/kg daily in divided doses
Cephazolin (Kefzol)	IM, IV or IVI 0.5–1 g every 6–12 hours; *child* 125–250 mg every 8 hours
Cephradine (Velasef)	IM, IV or IVI 0.5–1 g every 6 hours; *child* 50–100 mg/kg daily in 4 divided doses

Tetracyclines

Tetracycline (Achromycin)	IM 100–200 mg every 6–8 hours
	IVI 500 mg every 12 hours
Oxytetracycline	IM 100 mg every 8–12 hours
	Slow IV 250–500 mg every 12 hours

Aminoglycosides

Gentamicin (Cidomycin, Garamycin, Genticin)	IM 2–5 mg/kg daily in divided doses every 8 hours; in renal impairment the interval between successive doses should be increased to 12 hours when the creatinine clearance is 30–70 ml/min; 24 hours for 10–30 ml/min, 48 hours for 5–10 ml/min and 3–4 days after dialysis for less than 5 ml/min
	Child up to 2 weeks 3 mg/kg every 12 hours, 2 weeks–12 years 2 mg/kg every 8 hours
Amikacin (Amikin)	IM, IV 15 mg/kg daily in 2 divided doses
Kanamycin (Kannasyn)	IM 250 mg every 6 hours or 500 mg every 12 hours
	Slow IVI 15–30 mg/kg daily in divided doses every 8–12 hours
Tobramycin (Nebcin)	IM, IV or IVI 3–5 mg/kg daily in dividied doses every 8 hours

Table A.1 (*Cont.*)

Macrolides	
Erythromycin (Erythrocin)	IM 100 mg every 4–8 hours Slow IV or IVI 300 mg every 6 hours *or* 600 mg every 8 hours; *child* 30–50 mg/kg daily in divided doses every 6 hours
Other Antibiotics	
Clindamycin (Dalacin)	IM or slow IV 0.6–2.7 g daily in 2–4 divided doses; *child* 50–40 mg/kg daily in 3–4 divided doses
Lincomycin (Lincosin)	IM 600 mg every 12–24 hours
	Slow IV 600 mg every 8–12 hours
Chloramphenicol (Chloromycetin)	IV, IM 1 g every 6–8 hours; *child* pyogenic meningitis 500–100 mg/kg daily in divided doses every 6 hours; infants under 1 month 25 mg/kg daily in divided doses every 6 hours
Sodium fusidate (Fucidin)	Slow IV 500 mg over 6 hours, 3 times daily
Polymyxin B sulphate (Aerosporin)	Slow IVI 15 000–25 000 units/kg daily in divided doses
Antifungal drugs	
Amphotericin (Fungizone)	IVI 250 μg/kg daily gradually increased if tolerated to 1 mg/kg daily; maximum in severly ill patients 1.5 mg/kg daily or on alternate days
Flucytosine (Alcobon)	IVI 150–200 mg/kg daily in divided doses; reduce doses in renal impairment

Drugs affecting nutrition and blood

Heparin	1 mg $\equiv$ 100 i.u.
	IV 5000 i.u. followed by continuous infusion of 40 000 i.u. over 24 hours *or* 10 000 i.u. by IV injections every 6 hours
Warfarin (Marevan)	PO 10 mg daily for 3 days; maintenance usually 3–10 mg daily
Phenindione (Dindevan)	PO 200 mg on first day; 100 mg on second day; maintenance dose usually 50–150 mg daily
Nicoumalone (Sinthrome)	PO 8–10 mg on first day; 4–12 mg on second day; maintenance dose usually 1–6 mg daily
Aminocaproic acid (Epsikapron)	PO 3 g 4–6 times daily
Tranexamic acid (Cyclokapron)	PO 1 g 3–4 times daily Slow IV 1–2 g 3 times daily

Table A.1 (*Cont.*)

Aprotinin (Trasylol)	For acute pancreatitis and disseminated intravascular coagulation:
	Slow IV 500 000 kallidinogenase (Kallikrein) inactivator units, then 200 000 units by IVI every 4 hours
Sodium bicarbonate	Used in treatment of metabolic acidosis:
	Slow IV 4.2–8.4% solution *or* IVI a weak solution usually 1.4% to correct body base deficit
	(1 ml of 8.4% contains 1 mmol bicarbonate)
Potassium chloride	To correct potassium deficiency:
	IV concentration of solutions should not exceed 3.2 g (43 mmol/l).
	Slow IVI up to 6 g (80 mmol) daily
Calcium gluconate	Cardiac arrest:
	IV 10 ml calcium gluconate 10%
Calcium chloride	
(a) Anhydrous, $CaCl_2$	10% solution contains 0.91 mmol/ml
(b) Dihydrate, $CaCl_2.2H_2O$	13.4% solution contains 0.91 mmol/ml
(c) Hexahydrate, $CaCl_2.6H_2O$	20% solution contains 0.91 mmol/ml (i.e. these three different strengths contain about 1 mmol/ml)
Vitamins	
Vitamin K, Phytomenadione (Konakion)	IM or slow IV 10–20 mg as an antidote to oral anticoagulant drugs; maximum dose 40 mg IV in 24 hours

Drugs acting on the kidney and liver

Mannitol injection	10% or 20% solution
	IVI 50–200 g over 24 hours, preceded by a test dose of 200 mg/kg by slow IV
Frusemide (Lasix)	IM or slow IV 20–50 mg; *child* 0.5–1.5 mg/kg
	IVI in oliguria, 0.25–1 g at rate not exceeding 4 mg/min
Ethacrynic acid (Edecrin)	Slow IV or IVI 50 mg
Bumetanide (Burinex)	IM or IV 0.5–2 mg
	IVI 2–5 mg over 30–60 minutes

Muscle relaxant drugs

These must never be given to any patient who is not receiving adequate mechanical lung ventilation. Pancuronium is the drug of choice in intensive care as it does not cause significant histamine release or significant changes in blood pressure; there is no evidence that it causes ganglionic blockade

Table A.1 (*Cont.*)

Pancuronium bromide (Pavulon)	IV 60 μg/kg every $1-1\frac{1}{2}$ hours IM 30–60 μg every 1–2 hours
Suxamethonium chloride	IV 20–100 mg for tracheal intubation; *child* 1–1.5 mg/kg

Drugs acting on the endocrine system

Short-acting insulin preparation	Soluble insulin injection (acid, about pH 3.2, of mixed beef and pork origin) Neutral insulin injection (neutral pH and highly purified monospecies insulins)
Glucagon	Used to treat acute hypoglycaemic reactions: SC, IM, IV I mg dose (= 1 unit)
Corticosteroids	Replacement therapy: Addison's disease or after adrenalectomy, hydrocortisone 20–30 mg or cortisone acetate 25–37.5 mg daily by mouth, in 2 doses, the larger in the morning to mimic the normal diurnal rhythm of cortisol secretion Acute adrenocortical insufficiency: Hydrocortisone sodium succinate IV 100 mg every 6–8 hours in NaCl IV infusion Prednisone sodium phosphate injection is an alternative preparation for IV or IM use Dexamethasone: IM, IV or IVI 0.5–10 mg daily. Used in cases of cerebral oedema and after cardiac arrest. NB 1.3 mg dexamethasone phosphate = 1 mg dexamethasone

Appendix II

Emergency trays

1 In the Intensive Care Unit, the following equipment should be immediately available by the patient:
   (a) **Intubation tray** containing:
      Plastic cuffed endotracheal tubes, various sizes (with connectors)
      2 laryngoscopes (spare batteries and bulbs)
      1 endotracheal tube introducer
      1 catheter mount and connector
      1 rubber face mask and angle connector
      Airways of various sizes
      1 10 ml syringe (for inflating cuff of tube)
      1 pair artery forceps
      1 pair Magill's forceps
      1 length of $\frac{1}{2}''$ white tape
      1 tube of lubricating jelly
      Scissors
   (b) Equipment necessary for manual ventilation, attached to oxygen fitment
   (c) Equipment for tracheal suction

2 The following equipment should also be available in the unit:
   (a) **Resuscitation trolley** containing:
      A defibrillator with both adult and paediatric paddles
      Resuscitative drugs e.g. adrenaline, isoprenaline, calcium and sodium bicarbonate
      Equipment necessary for insertion of intravenous infusions
      A selection of syringes and needles
      Cardiac needles
      Mediswabs (sterile prepacked individual antiseptic swabs)
      Scissors and files
      Electrode jelly
   (b) O_2 masks and tubing for the giving of both medium concentration and venturi masks for fixed concentration oxygen therapy
   (c) A tracheostomy set and a selection of tracheostomy tubes
   (d) A bronchoscopy set
   (e) An ECG machine, patient cable and leads

3 A tracheostomy tray should also be available in the unit, containing:
   5 Cross action towel clips (Shardles)
   2 No 3 BP handles with No. 11 and No. 10 blades

1 $7\frac{1}{2}''$ curved scissors (McIndoe)
1 $6\frac{1}{2}''$ curved scissors (Mayo)
1 $4\frac{1}{2}''$ straight scissors (Iris)
2 6″ box joint forceps (Spencer Wells Artery)
2 6″ curved forceps (Spencer Wells Artery)
2 $1\frac{3}{4}'' \times 1\frac{1}{2}''$ retractors (Langenbeck)
2 double/blunt tracheostomy hooks
1 single/blunt tracheostomy hook
1 single/sharp tracheostomy hook
1 7″ non-toothed forceps (Waughs)
1 7″ toothed 1:2 forceps (Waughs)
1 5″ toothed 1:2 forceps (Treves)
1 8″ needle holder (Mayo)
1 suction tube (Gillies)
1 tracheal dilator (Bowlby)
1 2″ Gallipot
1 14 FG rubber suction catheter
10 4″ × 4″ radio-opaque gauze squares
10 2″ × 2″ gauze squares
5 pledgets
6 linen preparation towels
1 441 Ethicon (skin sutures)

Wrapping Method for sterilisation
Pulp tray (30.5 cm × 23 cm)
paper (100 × 100 cm)
paper bag (Code M)

Appendix III

Units, symbols and abbreviations

Approximate Conversions and Units

pounds	kilograms	stones	kilograms
1	0.45	1	6.35
2	0.91	2	12.70
3	1.36	3	19.05
4	1.81	4	25.40
5	2.27	5	31.75
6	2.72	6	38.10
7	3.18	7	44.45
8	3.63	8	50.80
9	4.08	9	57.15
10	4.54	10	63.50
11	4.99	11	69.85
12	5.44	12	76.20
13	5.90	13	82.55
14	6.35	14	88.90
		15	95.25
		16	101.60

ml	fluid ounces
50	1.8
100	3.5
150	5.3
200	7.0
250	8.8
300	10.6
350	12.4
400	14.0
450	15.8
500	17.6
1000	35.2

Mass

1 kilogram (kg)	= 1000 grams (g) (= 2.2 pounds).
1 gram (g)	= 1000 milligrams (mg)
1 milligram (mg)	= 1000 micrograms (μg)
1 microgram (μg)	= 1000 nanograms (ng)
1 nanogram (ng)	= 1000 picograms (pg)

Volume

1 litre (l)	= 1000 millilitres (ml)
1 millilitre (ml)	= 1000 microlitres (μl)
1 pint	= 568.3 ml
1 gallon	= 4.54609 l

Energy units

1 calorie (cal)	= 4.1868 joules (J)
1 kilocalorie (kcal)	= 4186.8 joules (J)
1000 kilocalories	= 4.1868 megajoules (MJ)

Pressure units

1 millimetre of mercury (mmHg)	= 133.3 pascals (Pa)
1 millimetre of mercury (mmHg)	= 0.735 centimetres of water (cmH_2O)
1 kilopascal (kPa)	= 7.5 mmHg

Primary Units

SI Unit	Quantity	Traditional metric unit
kilogram (kg)	mass	gram (g)
meter (m)	length	meter (m)
second (s)	time	second (s)
ampere (A)	electrical current	ampere (A)
kelvin (°K)	temperature	centigrade or Celsius (°C)
candela (Cd)	luminous intensity	lux (lx) (= lumen/m^2)
mole (mol)	amount of substance	milligram (mg), or milliequivalent (mEq)

Some Derived Units

cubic meter (m^3)	volume	litre (l)
Newton (N)	force	dyne
pascal (Pa)	pressure	mmHg, cmH_2O
joule (J)	work or energy	calorie (cal)
Watt (W)	power	watt (w)
Hertz (Hz)	periodic frequency	cycles/s

Prefixes for SI Units

Factor	Name	Symbol
10^{12}	tera-	T
10^9	giga-	G
10^6	mega-	M
10^3	kilo-	k
10^2	hecto-	h
10^1	deca-	da

Factor	Name	Symbol
10^{-1}	deci-	d
10^{-2}	centi-	c
10^{-3}	milli-	m
10^{-6}	micro-	μ
10^{-9}	nano-	n
10^{-12}	pico-	p
10^{-15}	femto-	f
10^{-18}	atto-	a

Although the official SI unit of volume is the cubic metre (m^3) the litre ($10^{-3}m^3 = dm^3$) is so convenient for clinical purposes that it is still used; 1 decilitre (dl) = 100 ml.

Some abbreviations used in respiratory physiology
(values in parentheses are for normal adult males)

Lung volume (litres)

TLC	total lung capacity (6000 ml)
VC	vital capacity (4800 ml)
IVC	inspiratory vital capacity
FRC	functional residual capacity (2400 ml)
IC	inspiratory capacity
ERV	expiratory reserve volume
RV	residual volume (1200 ml)

Ventilatory capacity

FEV	forced expiratory volume
$FEV_{1.0}$	forced expiratory volume over the first second
FVC	forced vital capacity
FET	forced expiratory time
FEV%	i.e. (FEV/FVC) × 100 (85%)
PEFR	peak expiratory flow rate
FEF	forced expiratory flow
AWR	airway resistance
A-aD	alveolar-arterial tension difference (e.g. for O_2)
TF	transfer factor

Symbols and Units

(*a*) *Primary symbols*
These are printed in italics. Fundamental quantities are volume (V), pressure (P), time (t) and amount of substance such as the number of moles. Volume per unit time ($V \div t$) is $\dot{V}$ in the gas phase and $\dot{Q}$ in the blood phase.

V = volume of gas or blood
$\dot{V}$ = gas volume per unit time
$\dot{Q}$ = blood volume per unit time (e.g. $\dot{Q}$ may represent cardiac output, litres/minute)
P = pressure
S = per cent saturation of haemoglobin with oxygen

(b) *Suffixes*

I	Inspired gas
E	expired gas
A	alveolar gas
T	tidal gas
D	deadspace gas
B	barometer pressure
a	arterial blood
v	venous blood
$\bar{v}$	mixed venous blood (i.e. pulmonary artery blood)
c	pulmonary capillary blood
c′	end-pulmonary capillary blood
va	venous admixture
pl	plasma

(c) *Examples*

V_T	tidal volume
V_D	deadspace volume
PA_{O_2}	pressure of oxygen in alveolar gas
Sa_{O_2}	arterial oxygen saturation
Pa_{O_2}	pressure of oxygen in arterial blood
$P\bar{v}_{O_2}$	pressure of oxygen in mixed venous blood
V_E	volume expired gas
V_A	alveolar ventilation
F_{ECO_2}	fractional concentration of CO_2 in the expired gas (e.g. $F_{ECO_2} = 0.03$ means 3% CO_2 in expired gas).
F_{IO_2}	fractional concentration of O_2 in the inspired gas

Appendix IV

Common normal values

(values vary slightly between laboratories)

1 Blood

General

Blood volume 5–6 litres (adult); 75 ml/kg body weight; 3 l/m² body surface area

Osmolarity (serum) 275–300 mOsm/l

Cardiac output 5–5.5 l/min at rest; in strenuous exercise up to 25 l/min (or more in athletes).

Cardiac Index 2.5–3.5 l/min/m²

Coronary circulation: about 250 ml/min at rest; flows may increase up to 1200 ml/min in maximal heart activity

Right atrial (RA) pressure (mean) 1.5 mmHg (0.2 kPa)

Pulmonary capillary wedge pressure (PCWP) (mean) 6–12 mmHg (0.8–1.6 kPa)

Pulmonary artery (PA) pressure 25 mmHg (3.3 kPa) systolic, 10 mmHg (1.3 kPa) diastolic

Haemoglobin 12–16 g/100 ml blood (variation for sex and age)

Red blood cells 4.5–6.0 million per mm³

Packed Cell Volume (PCV), men   40–54%

women   36–47%

Mean Corpuscular Haemoglobin Concentration (MCHC) 32–36 g/dl

Reticulocytes 0.2–2% of red cells

White blood cells (adult) total count $4–10 \times 10^9$/l

Neutrophils	40–75%
Lymphocytes	20–45%
Monocytes	2–10%
Eosinophils	1–6%
Basophils	0–1%
Platelets	$150–400 \times 10^9$/l

Chemical and physical properties

pH arterial blood 7.36–7.44

pH venous blood 7.34–7.42

Oxygen content of arterial blood 18–22 ml/100 ml blood

Carbon dioxide content of arterial blood 48–50 ml/100 ml blood

Arterial oxygen tension (P_{O_2}) 95–100 mmHg (12.67–13.33 kPa)

Arterial carbon dioxide tension ($P\text{co}_2$) 36–44 mmHg (4.8–5.87 kPa)
Oxygen content of venous blood 15–16 ml/100 ml
Carbon dioxide content of venous blood 52–54 ml/100 ml
Venous blood oxygen tension 37–42 mmHg (4.93–5.60 kPa)
Venous blood carbon dioxide tension 42–48 mmHg (5.60–6.40 kPa)
Standard bicarbonate 22–26 mmol/l
Actual bicarbonate 22–26 mmol/l
Buffer Base 47–49 mmol/l
Osmolality 275–295 mOsmol/kg
Base Excess +2.5 to −2.5 mmol/l
Circulation time, arm to tongue 9–16 s
Bleeding time, Duke's method, 2–5 min
     Ivy, Nelson and Butcher, 3 min (max. 4 min)
Coagulation time, capillary, 10–15 min; venous, 3–7 min
Sedimentation rate (Westergren) Men 1 h, 7–12 mm
         Women 1 h, 10–18 mm
Glucose (fasting) 3.3–6.7 mmol/l
 normal renal threshold 10 mmol/l
Urea 3.0–7.0 mmol/l

Plasma Electrolytes

Inorganic Ions (serum):
 Sodium 135–150 mmol/l
 Potassium 3.5–5.6 mmol/l
 Calcium 2.2–2.5 mmol/l
 Chlorides 96–106 mmol/l
 Magnesium 0.7–1.0 mmol/l
 Phosphate, adults 0.8–1.4 mmol/l
     children 1.3–1.9 mmol/l
Cholesterol (total) 3.6–7.2 mmol/l
Fibrinogen (plasma) 2–4 g/l
Lactic acid (blood) 6–16 mg/100 ml
Pyruvic acid (plasma) 1–2 mg/100 ml
Serum protein, Total 60–70 g/l
    Albumin 35–55 g/l
    Globulin 25–30 g/l
Bilirubin 6–20 μmol/l
Urea 3.0–7.0 mmol/l
Pseudocholinesterase 60–90 Warburg units
Serum bilirubin 5–17 μmol/l
Bromsulphthalein liver function (2 mg/kg); less than 5 % of dye should
 remain after 45 minutes
Thymol turbidity less than 4 units
Alkaline phosphatase (King and Armstrong) 4–14 KA units (up to 20
 units in children)

Acid phosphatase (Gutman and Gutman) up to 5 KA units
Creatinine in plasma 60–120 μmol/l
Creatinine clearance more than 60 ml/min
Diastatic index (serum) 2–15 Wohlgemuth units

2 Urine

Volume 600–2500 ml/24 hours (average 1200 ml)
pH 4.8–7.4 (average 6.0)
Specific gravity (SG) 1.010–1.025
Sodium 100–250 mmol/l
Potassium 40–120 mmol/l
Chlorides 4–10 g (100–300 mmol)
Calcium 2.5–7.5 mmol/24 h
Urea 250–500 mmol/l
Creatinine 9–17 mmol/24 h
Ammonia 0.3–1 g/24 h
Uric acid 0.12–0.42 mmol/l
Protein 0.01 g
Amylase (diastase) 8–32 units
Osmolility 30–1400 mOsmol/kg

3 Cerebrospinal fluid (CSF)

pH 7.32–7.35
Pressure 100–130 mm CSF (10–13 cmH$_2$O)
Cells < 5 × 10^9/l
Calcium 0.6–0.65 mmol/l
Chloride 130–128 mmol/l
Potassium 2.4–3.2 mmol/l
Sodium 140–150 mmol/l
Bicarbonate 23 mmol/l
Glucose 1.5–4.0 mmol/l
Protein (total) 24–40 mg/100 ml
Urea 10–30 mg/100 ml

4 Secretions (volume/day)

Saliva 1500 ml
Gastric juice 2–3 litres (pH 0.9–1.5)
Bile 500–1000 ml
Pancreatic juice 500–800 ml
Succus entericus 3000 ml
Insensible loss 400 ml
Normal stool 200 ml

5 *Fluid compartments*

Total body water 45 litres
Extracellular space 12–15 litres
Intracellular space 25–30 litres
Interstitial space 9 litres

Example of normal fluid balance

All volumes are approximate and will depend upon environmental
conditions, diet and exercise taken.

in		*out*	
Water from solids	700 ml	Skin (insensible loss)	500 ml
Water from oxidation	300 ml	Lungs	400 ml
Fluids by mouth	1500 ml	Faeces	100 ml
		Urine	1500 ml
Total	2500 ml	Total	2500 ml

Appendix V

Suggested further reading

ADAMS, A. P., HAHN, C. E. W. (1982). *Principles and Practice of Blood-Gas Analysis* 2nd Edn. Churchill Livingstone, London.

BECK, J. S. (Ed). (1975). Symposium on a Physiological Approach to Critical Care. *Surgical Clinics of North America, 55, 3, June.*

BOLD, A. M., WILDING, P. (1978). *Clinical Chemistry Companion.* Blackwell Scientific Publications.

CAMPKIN, T. V., TURNER, J. M. (1980). *Neurosurgical Anaesthesia and Intensive Care.* Butterworths, London.

COTES, J. E. (1979). *Lung Function: Assessment and Application in Medicine* 4th Edn. Blackwell Scientific Publications.

CROFTON, J., DOUGLAS, A. (1981). *Respiratory Diseases.* Blackwell Scientific Publications.

DUNNILL, R. P. H., CRAWLEY, B. E. (1977). *Clinical and Resuscitative Data.* Blackwell Scientific Publications.

GOLDBERGER, E. (1982). *A Primer of Water, Electrolytes and Acid-Base Syndromes.* Lea and Febiger, Philadelphia.

JOHNSTON, I. D. A (Ed). (1978). *Advances in Parenteral Nutrition.* MPT Press, Lancaster.

LEDINGHAM, I. McA., HANNING, C. D. (1983). *Recent Advances in Critical Care Medicine—2.* Churchill-Livingstone, London.

McPHERSON, S. P. (1981). *Respiratory Therapy Equipment* 2nd Edn. C: V. Mosby, St. Louis.

NUNN, J. F. (1977). *Applied Respiratory Physiology* 2nd Edn. Butterworths, London.

OPIE, L. H. (1980). *Drugs and the Heart.* The Lancet.

PALLIS, C. (1983). *ABC of Brain Stem Death.* British Medical Journal Publications, London.

RUSSELL, W. J. (1974). *Central Venous Pressure: Its Clinical Use and Role in Cardiovascular Dynamics.* Butterworths, London.

SYKES, M. K., McNICOL, M. W., CAMPBELL, E. J. M. (1976). *Respiratory Failure* 2nd Edn. Blackwell Scientific Publications.

TINKER, J., RAPIN, M. (Eds). (1983). *Care of the Critically Ill Patient.* Springer-Verlag, Berlin.

WEST, J. B. (1977). *Pulmonary Pathophysiology: The Essentials.* Blackwell Scientific Publications.

WEST, J. B. (1979). *Respiratory Physiology: The Essentials.* Blackwell Scientific Publications.

WILLATTS, S. M. (1982). *Lecture Notes on Fluid and Electrolyte Balance.* Blackwell Scientific Publications.

Papers on 'brain death' and 'removal of cadaveric organs for transplantation':

1 Conference of Medical Royal Colleges and their Faculties in the United Kingdom. *The Lancet, 1976, ii, 1069–70.*

2 Conference of Medical Royal Colleges and their Faculties in the United Kingdom. *The British Medical Journal, 1976, ii, 1187–8.*

3 Conference of Medical Royal Colleges and their Faculties in the United Kingdom. *The Lancet, 1979, i, 261–2.*

4 Conference of Medical Royal Colleges and their Faculties in the United Kingdom. *The British Medical Journal, 1979, i, 332.*

5 The Removal of Cadaveric Organs for Transplantation: A Code of Practice. *Health Departments of Great Britain and Northern Ireland. HMSO, London, (1979).*

6 Brain Death. J. G. Robson. *The British Medical Journal, 1981, 283, 5050.*

Appendix VI

Record charts used in the intensive care unit

BLOOD BALANCE SHEET

RECORD No.

NAME ....

SHEET NUMBER ....

BALANCE ON RETURN ....

TIME	DRAINAGE TUBES LEFT				RIGHT			TOTAL OUT	BLOOD ETC. IN	BALANCE	HOURLY DRAINAGE TOTAL	REMARKS

Sheet No.

GUY'S HOSPITAL INTENSIVE TREATMENT UNIT

OBSERVATION CHART

SURNAME .... OTHER NAMES .... AGE .... CONSULTANT .... UNIT No. .... HEIGHT .... WEIGHT .... SURFACE AREA ....

DATE

TIME

TEMPERATURES

41
40	300
39	290
38	280
37	270
36	260
35	250
34	240
33	230
32	220
31	210
30	200
29	190
28	180
27	170
26	160
25	150
24	140
23	130
22	120
21	110
20	100
	90
APEX	80
B/P	70
V/P	60
L/A	50
	40
	30
	20
	10

PULSES	L
	R
RHYTHM	
CONTINUOUS INFUSIONS	
DROPS/MIN.	
RELEVANT DRUGS	
PRESS. insp. 80	
PEEP/CPAP 75	
VOL. pre set 70	
measured 65	
patient 60	
55	
RATE IPPV/IMV 50	
patient 45	
insp. time 40	
exp. time 35	
30	
25	
INSP. TEMP. 20	
ENTONOX 15	
AIR 10	
OXYGEN 5	
Per cent. O₂	
Turning	
P/Areas	
Suction	
Cuff Check	
T. Dressing	
Eye Care	
Oral Toilet	
Leg Exs.	
Cath. Toilet	
REMARKS	

GUY'S HOSPITAL INTENSIVE TREATMENT UNIT

CHART II

Sheet No.................................. NAME.................................. WARD.................................. UNIT NO..................................

	DATE																		
	DAY																		
	Time:																		
	Na																		
B	K																		
L	HCO₃																		
O	Urea																		
O	Osmo																		
D	Creatinine																		
	Glucose																		
	Time:																		
	Hb.																		
	P.C.V.																		
	W.B.C.																		
	Platelets																		
	K.C.T.																		
	P.T.																		
	T.T.																		
	Fib. Titre																		
	Time:																		
	Na.																		
U	K.																		
R	Urea																		
I	Osmo																		
N	Creatinine																		
E																			
	Time:																		
	pH																		
	PCO₂																		
	PO₂																		
B G	**SHCO₃**																		
L A	B.Excess																		
O S	Vent.																		
O E	%O₂																		
D S	PEEP/CPAP																		
	I.M.V.																		
	Time:																		
L																			
D E																			
R V																			
U E																			
G L																			
S																			

Ward/Clinic			Consultant		**GUY'S HEALTH DISTRICT**

Surname
First Name
Date of Birth
Address

Unit No.

Sex

NEUROLOGICAL OBSERVATION CHART

Sheet No:

Bed No:			Date :	
			Time	
C O M	EYES OPEN (Eyes closed by swelling = C)		Spontaneously	
			To speech	
			To pain	
			None	
A S C	BEST VERBAL RESPONSE (Intubated = T)		Orientated	
			Confused	
			Inappropriate Words	
			Incomprehensible Sounds	
			None	
A L E	BEST MOTOR RESPONSE (Better arm)		Obey commands	
			Localise pain	
			Flexion to pain	
			Extension to pain	
			None	

Pupil scale (mm): dots sized 1 through 8

Temperature °C / Blood pressure and Pulse rate / Respiration rate

41 240
40 230
39 220
38 210
37 200
36 190
35 180
34 170
33 160
32 150
31 140
30 130
120
110
100
90
80
70
60
50
40
30
20
10

PUPILS (C = eye closed)	R	Size Reaction (+ or −)	
	L	Size Reaction (+ or −)	

L I M B M O V E M E N T	A R M S	Normal power	
		Mild weakness	
		Severe weakness	
		Spastic flexion	
		Extension	
		No response	
	L E G S	Normal power	
		Mild weakness	
		Severe weakness	
		Extension	
		No response	

Record Right with black spot, Left with open circle if different

See over for guidance notes

Appendix VII

National Poisons Information Service

	Telephone Number
London (Co-ordinating Centre at Guy's Hospital)	01 407 7600
Belfast	0232 240503
Cardiff	0222 569200
Edinburgh	031 229 2477
Dublin	0001 745588

(These telephone numbers were correct at the time of going to press).

Index